Knowledge to Care

A Handbook for Care Assistants

Knowledge to Care

A Handbook for Care Assistants

Second Edition

Edited by

Angela Dustagheer
MA Educ (London), Dip Ed, RN, RNT

Joan Harding
MA, BA, RN, RM, RNT

Christine McMahon
TD, RGN, BSc, RONT, TNT

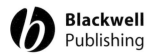
Blackwell
Publishing

© First edition 1994 Christine A. McMahon & Joan Harding
© Second edition 2005 by Blackwell Publishing Ltd

Editorial offices:
Blackwell Publishing Ltd, 9600 Garsington Road, Oxford OX4 2DQ, UK
  Tel: +44 (0)1865 776868
Blackwell Publishing Inc., 350 Main Street, Malden, MA 02148-5020, USA
  Tel: +1 781 388 8250
Blackwell Publishing Asia Pty Ltd, 550 Swanston Street, Carlton, Victoria 3053, Australia
  Tel: +61 (0)3 8359 1011

First edition published 1993 by Blackwell Science Ltd
Second edition published 2005 by Blackwell Publishing Ltd

Library of Congress Cataloging-in-Publication Data
Knowledge to care : a handbook for care assistants / edited by Angela Dustagheer, Joan Harding, Christine McMahon. – 2nd ed.
    p.; cm.
  Includes bibliographical references and index.
  ISBN 1-4051-1111-9 (pbk. : alk. paper)
    1. Nurses' aides.   2. Care of the sick.   3. Nursing.
  [DNLM: 1. Nurses' Aides.   2. Nursing Care – methods. WY 193 K73 2004]
  I. Dustagheer, Angela.   II. Harding, Joan.   III. McMahon, Christine A.

RT84.K57 2004
610.73'06'98 – dc22
                                                      2004011389

ISBN   1-4051-1111-9

A catalogue record for this title is available from the British Library

Set in 10 on 12.5 pt Palatino
by SNP Best-set Typesetter Ltd., Hong Kong
Printed and bound in India
by Gopsons Papers Ltd., New Delhi

The publisher's policy is to use permanent paper from mills that operate a sustainable forestry policy, and which has been manufactured from pulp processed using acid-free and elementary chlorine-free practices. Furthermore, the publisher ensures that the test paper and cover board used have met acceptable environmental accreditation standards.

For further information on Blackwell Publishing, visit our website:
www.blackwellpublishing.com

Contents

*Contributor to the original version of this chapter in the first edition.

List of contributors

Elizabeth Atchison*, MSc, RGN, RNT, Cert Ed, Formerly Senior Lecturer (Macmillan), School of Acute Care, University of Luton, Luton and Dunstable Hospital, Luton

Caroline Coleman, RNMH, Cert in Adult/Further Education, Diploma in Management Studies, Unit Manager, Adult Services, Hertfordshire County Council

Patricia Cronin, Dip N (Lond), BSc Nursing and Education, MSc Nursing, RN, Senior Lecturer, Adult Nursing, St Bartholomew School of Nursing and Midwifery, City University, London

Katie Cullinan, MSc, Reg MRCSLT, Specialist Speech and Language Therapist, UCLH NHS Trust, London

Angela Dustagheer, MA Educ (Lond), Dip Ed, RN, RNT, Advanced Dip Counselling/Interpersonal Skills, ENB N37 Palliative Care, TDLB: D32, 33, 34, 36, BTEC Management NVQ Level 5/Lecturer Practioner based at UCLH NHS Trust, London

Christine Ely, MSc, BA, RN, RM, Cert Ed, Lecturer in Nurse Education, City University, London

Chris Flatt, BSc (Hons) Nutrition, State Registered Dietitian, Chief Dietitian, Queen Mary's Hospital, Roehampton, London

Sandra Fortuna, Licentiate's Degree in Clinical Psychology, PgD Dramatherapy, RDth, MPC Membership Chartered in Clinical Psychology; Full Membership BPS, Chartered Clinical Psychologist, Hertfordshire Partnership NHS Disabilities Trust, St Albans Learning Services, Herts

Rita Gale, City & Guilds, 9292 (Staff Assessors Award), 9294 (Direct Training & Assessors Award), 7281/12 (Vocational Assessors Award), Licentiate of the Institute of Health Record Information & Management, Independent Health Records Consultant

Frank Garvey, BA (Hons), RMNH, RGN, RNT, Cert Ed, Cert Health Ed, ENB 998, ENB N45, Senior Community Learning Disability Nurse, Dacorum, Hertfordshire Partnership Trust

Karen Gillett, Msc, BSc (Hons), RGN, PG Dip Nursing (Ed), Lecturer in Cancer Nursing, St Bartholomew School of Nursing/Midwifery, City University, London

Joan Harding, MA, BA, RN, RM, RNT, Independent Nurse Consultant

Hazel Heath, MSc, BA (Hons), RGN, RCNT, RNT, Dip N (Lond), FETC, Cert Ed, ITEC Independent Nurse Consultant, Editor of *Nursing Older People*, Nurse Advisor to Elizabeth Finn Trust

Christine McMahon*, TD, RGN, BSc, Dip N (Lond), RCNT, Dip N Ed (Lond), RNT, Formerly Vocational Qualifications Consultant

Jenny Partridge, BSc (Hons), RGN, Dip N (Lond), PG CEA, MBA, MIHM, Senior Tutor, European Institute of Health and Medical Sciences, University of Surrey, Guildford

Lynne Phair, MA, BSc (Hons), DPNS, PG Cert RMN, RGN, Advanced Cert Health & Safety, Consultant Nurse Older People, Crawley Primary Care Trust

Fay Reid, BA, RN, Dip N (Lond), RNT, MSc, Cert in Personnel Management, Back Care & Manual Handling Consultant

Heather Rowe, RGN, BA, RCNT, Dip N (Lond), Principal Lecturer, Faculty of Health Studies, Buckinghamshire Chilterns University College

Dorothy Stables*, MSc, BA (Hons), RGN, RM, Dip N (Lond), MTD, Senior Midwife Teacher/Course Director, St Bartholomew's College of Nursing and Midwifery, London

Rebecca Sutton, Dip Higher Education (Midwifery), Midwife, Elizabeth Garrett Anderson and Obstetric Hospital, UCLH, London

Judith Trendall, MSc, BA (Hons), RGN, RNT, Lecturer in Adult Nursing, St Bartholomew School of Nursing/Midwifery City University, London

Jane Watson née Powell*, BSc (Hons), Dip in Dietetics, Assessor Award (D32/33), Chief Community Dietitian

Lisa S. Whiting, BA (Hons), MSc, RGN, RSCN, RNT, LTCL, Senior Lecturer, Children's Nursing, University of Hertfordshire, Hatfield, Herts

*Contributor to first edition of 'Knowledge to Care'

Foreword: knowledge to care second edition

Anthony Palmer, RGN, DPSN, BSc(Hons), PGCEA
Director of Nursing, Royal National Orthopaedic Hospital, Brockley Hill, Stanmore

The healthcare Assistant (HCA) role is rapidly expanding and increasing in responsibility as they take on more of the burden of direct care in clinical areas to support the registered nurse, whose role is also expanding and diversifying to take on more of the doctor's work. In order to do this the health carer is required to deliver a high standard of care within the multi-disciplinary team. This second edition is a welcome text as there still remains a paucity of literature available specifically for HCAs and will provide a useful resource. It is not specifically written as an accompanying text to the NVQ Care Award but does remained focused to provide a text to cover the underpinning knowledge for the mandatory and some of the other NVQ Units. The NVQ Award continues to provide a mechanism to improve standards of care and to the work based competencies of the carers and thus contribute to the quality of patient care. Recently the Award has become increasingly seen as a vehicle for HCAs to access pre-registration nursing courses.

The authors and contributors to the second edition are clinical and educational experts in a diverse range of health care fields. Some chapters have been updated by the original contributors, others have been written by new chapter authors, however the effort has been made to maintain the continuity of the book. The text is not written in relation to tasks, rather it is orientated in a manner to include authentic and practical material to guide the HCA in their role and to provide a guide to the professional practioner who is working with the carers. Its central tenet is to highlight the importance of providing planned, holistic, patient centred care; giving a rationale for the care delivered.

It has attempted to provide a clear and easily understood text and the chapters have retained the format of including activities for readers to undertake, thus encouraging them to interact with the written material. The book should appeal to a wider audience than those undertaking the NVQ Care Award as it provides a major source of practical advice and support for all those engaged in patient care.

Editor's acknowledgements

We are grateful to all the contributors to this second edition. Their undoubted knowledge of and expertise in the topics about which they have written create a book of value to our readers to help them provide high quality care.

We would like to offer thanks to Anthony Palmer for writing the Foreword, to Lotika Singh for her patient assistance and valuable observations in preparing the manuscript. We would also express our appreciation of Matthew Smith for his skilled work in producing all the images for the book.

We are grateful to all the staff at Blackwell Publishing and in particular to Beth Knight who first suggested we undertake a second edition, kept us on track with the many tasks involved and encouraged us when spirits flagged, to ensure that the book finally emerged.

Finally we are indebted to families and friends who offered support and encouragement at the right moments and to David for providing many cups of coffee as work progressed.

To you all we say – Thank you.

Introduction
Who the book is for and how to use it

Joan Harding

Care is about using warmth, knowledge, understanding and skill to help another. Many have the capacity to care but lack the knowledge and skills to do so with confidence. *Knowledge to Care* aims to provide the knowledge base from which those skills and awareness can be developed and enable carers to feel confident about what they do and how they do it.

Caring is usually a group or team activity, which needs organisation and a leader. Care in health care settings will usually be directed by professional practitioners of various disciplines; therefore care assistants assist in care and are responsible to these professionals.

Scope of care for health care assistants

Over the past 10–15 years the development of the health care assistant role as a support to professional practitioners in various disciplines has been a vitally important element of the team approach to care, with significant implications for the quality of care delivered. It has also opened a whole range of training opportunities in vocational training for carers to ensure that quality care is maintained.

Health care assistants work under the direction and supervision of registered practitioners, who remain accountable for the standards of care delivered and for determining the activity of their support staff, which must not be beyond their level of competence.

However, it cannot be said too often that support given by individuals who have acquired skill through knowledge and training can only enhance the quality of care given to individual clients. Therefore, health care assistants should be encouraged and supported in obtaining vocational qualifications which recognise their skills, and these skills can be used for the benefit of their clients in a variety of settings. Looking to the future as the make-up of caring teams evolves and changes to meet requirements of the day, one can foresee the continued need for carers to undertake work-based training and attain appropriate qualifications.

We hope that this volume will be of value to:

Learners (care assistants): as a source of information to act as a starting point for increasing knowledge and skill

Teachers: as a resource in support of courses for health care assistants

Patients and clients: who will receive quality care from carers who have taken time to acquire knowledge and develop skills.

About this book

On first opening a book a number of questions spring to mind. The information below is to help you decide whether this is the book you are looking for.

What is the book about?
  It is about caring in health care settings.

Who is the book for?
  It is written for health care assistants, nurse cadets and those involved in caring in hospitals, nursing and residential homes, the community, or even looking after their own relatives or friends at home. *Knowledge to Care* is just that – it aims to provide information to help you understand the whys and wherefores of care for a range of patients or clients in a range of situations. Nurse cadets will find it helpful as an introduction to the care environment and to responding to clients as individuals with their own hopes, fears and anxieties.

Is it about exams, tests or qualifications?
  That is entirely up to you. If you are involved in preparing for assessment for NVQs (National Vocational Qualifications) the book will help you towards your goal. Alternatively, you may like to use it to enhance your understanding of the work you do each day. You may also find it helpful if you are involved in a caring course in a college or other institution.

How the book is presented

This second edition of *Knowledge to Care* is based on the format of the first one – the text has been revised and updated to reflect current health care practice.
  The book progresses from general subjects to those which are more specialised. Each chapter corresponds to specific parts of the framework of national care awards. Chapters 1–6 cover general principles which apply to most care settings; Chapters 7–13 deal with aspects of direct care and Chapters 14–17 cover care in a selection of more specific situations, e.g. postnatal, the young child and the terminally ill.
  The book is primarily concerned with care given in health care institutions, though the principles may be applied in a variety of settings. The contents link closely with units of competence as they appear in the National Occupational Standards for Care NVQ, level 2. As the book is intended for carers working in a variety of settings – what should we call those for whom we are caring? We decided to take the middle road so you will find the term 'client' is used most

often, but 'patient' or 'service user' also appear where it seems more appropriate to use that term. Perhaps by the time another edition is due we will all be using something else . . . !

Most chapters have some 'Key words' at the beginning. These provide a brief indication of the content of the chapter and, in particular, items or points to be remembered. These same words usually appear again as or in headings to sections of the chapter.

Activities

In most chapters you will find material in boxes with the heading 'Activity' followed by a number. Here you will be invited to stop and think, draw up a list, consider what you would do in certain circumstances, reflect on instances you have already encountered, or discuss a topic with a colleague or colleagues. The whole aim of these activities is to extend the range of material beyond the text of the chapter(s) and to encourage you to use your own thoughts, ideas or experiences. However, you may wish to read the chapter first and then return to the activities. There is no right or wrong way, whatever you decide to do is right for you.

Throughout the text you will find current day examples or short stories intended to help you remember certain items or facts. No doubt by the time you have finished the book, and as a result of your own experiences and those you share with your colleagues, you will surely expand the content beyond the original covers.

Finally, to help you locate the part of the book you most want at a particular time, the contents list includes the main heading in each chapter, a comprehensive index and an appendix for matching up items in the text with units of the National Occupational Standards for NVQs in Care.

Chapter 1
Clients' rights

Angela Dustagheer

Overview

This chapter provides an introduction to human rights, which are linked to entitlement, and should be incorporated into all policy and practice relating to clients' rights. These rights are embedded into good care delivery practices. Rights in care are not only related to meeting a client's needs but include the carer's involvement in enabling them to access services. As carers we have a responsibility to know about an individual's legal and personal rights. The chapter is divided into two sections: rights of clients and the delivery of care.

Key words: Human rights; clients' rights; legislation; core care values; responsibility; advocacy; diversity; equal opportunity; universal precautions; trust and confidentiality

Rights of clients

> There is no more vibrant, hope filled and complex idea alive in the world today than human rights and dignity for all.
>
> International Federation of Red Cross and Red Crescent Societies and
> François-Xavier Bagnoud Centre for Health and Human Rights [1]

Human rights underlie the core care values that underpin the concept of caring for others. As individual citizens we are entitled to basic rights, although these do vary depending on the country in which you live. There is an issue of responsibility, i.e. a human being has rights, governments/society has a responsibility to provide those rights and the individual is responsible for society's and others' rights. In relation to health, the government provides care but individuals should also take responsibility for their own health. Within organisations responsibility is encapsulated in staff policies and protocols and professionals operate within mutually agreed codes of conduct.

Activity 1.1

Make a list of all the rights you believe you have and which you can access. You can discuss your list with another person or in a group. Write down everything that is said.

Your list will probably contain some of the following:

* Right to legal representation
* Right to vote
* Right to free primary and secondary school education
* Right to health care free at the point of delivery
* Right to freedom of speech
* Right to freedom of movement

Health care is delivered and operates within a framework of legislation, regulations, policies and procedures. These determine how work is carried out. It is important that you know of the existence of information on this legislation and the implications for care within your organisation. Remember that your client has citizens' rights.

The following are some of the more important Acts and regulations which address human rights issues:

* Universal Declaration of Human Rights 1948[2]
* Declaration on Rights of Mentally Retarded Persons 1971[3]
* Health and Safety Act 1974[4]
* Sex Discrimination Act 1975[5]
* Race Relations Discrimination Act 1976[6]
* Mental Health Acts 1983[7,8]
* Disabled Persons Act 1986[9]
* Children Act 1989[10,11]
* Community Care Act 1990[12]
* Food Safety Act 1990[13]
* Disability Discrimination Act 1995[14]
* Data Protection Act 1998[15]
* Public Interest Disclosure Act 1998[16]
* Human Rights Act 1998[17]
* Care Standards Act 2000[18]

The Human Rights Act 1998 is the most recent legislation and may prove to be a major trigger to the way care is delivered.

Activity 1.2

Where would you find information regarding rights?
  You would need to check out:

- Codes of practice
- Professional codes of conduct
- Staff policies
- Policies for service users
- Guidelines or standards of care
- Clients' individual care plans

  Your answer may also include

- Citizen's advice bureaux
- Libraries
- Internet

In the National Health Service (NHS) the *Patient's Charter* is used as a philosophy of care. The *Patient's Charter* was produced by the Department of Health (DoH) in 1991[19,20]. The document includes clients' rights to care as well as the standard of service. The values outlined in the *Patient's Charter* include: health care is free at the point of delivery, and emergency medical care is available at all times to everyone.

The charter also includes details regarding provision of local health services, including quality of provision and waiting times. Everyone has the right to be registered with a general practitioner (GP) and if necessary receive a referral to a consultant/specialist, and to have a second opinion. In addition, everyone must have a guaranteed admission date (two years from the time they were placed on the waiting list). Informed consent is a right: each person must be given an explanation regarding the proposed treatment including problems, risks and possible alternatives and this should be done prior to treatment. Confidentiality is a right and everyone should have access to his or her own records. All NHS complaints should be investigated promptly, and the complainant should receive a written reply. The client also has the right to choose whether to be involved in medical student training and medical research and has the right to opt out at any time.

Diversity

Each client is a unique individual with a personal biography; the majority of people are surrounded by a family and/or those significant to them and to whom she or he relates. The individual will have been socialised through her or his family, schooling and amongst friends and the wider culture; thus she or he will have a set of beliefs, customs and behaviours. In the UK, we are a pluralistic (multi-cultural) society and therefore people may have different, even contrasting, life views and lifestyles. As carers, we should recognise, and be aware of, the many different life worlds and we have a responsibility to incorporate this diversity into care and ensure that people's beliefs, customs and mores are not infringed and also ensure that the client is helped to meet their needs. Our aim should be to empower individuals. In order to do this, it is necessary to listen effectively and be aware of our limitations. This requires good communication, and interpersonal and interaction skills. We need to be clear in our speech and use of language, avoiding jargon and abbreviations and taking time to listen to people so that they can express their concerns and issues. This aspect is dealt with in more detail in Chapter 4 (Communication).

Equal opportunity

Care delivery should reflect an equal opportunity approach, and an anti-discriminatory care practice is to be actively promoted. Every person has the right to be seen as a unique individual who has a personal biography and social history which needs to be recognised and incorporated into his or her plan of care. The issues relating to ethics, cultural differences and difficult dilemmas in care are discussed in Chapter 2.

Everybody involved in care should take personal responsibility to ensure a good standard of care is delivered and should be able to raise any concern regarding standards of care. This involves protecting the vulnerable person, being alert to the signs of abuse and reporting any concerns to management. This may be a difficult position to be in, especially if the clients' rights are not met, or are stopped when linked to insufficient resources, which could be related to issues of funding staff and equipment.

Activity 1.3

If you were to draft a patient's charter, what rights would you include? Make a list of clients' rights and compare and discuss your list with someone else involved in care. Are they the same? How do they differ?

Your answer may include the right to:

- Personal privacy, independence
- Personal dignity
- Self care
- Refuse treatment and care
- Have access to and/or have help to access their GP, member of Parliament, family and significant others
- Be involved in drawing up the plan of care
- Have religious, cultural and sexual orientation accepted/respected

Certain principles of care and core care values have arisen from the matrix of legislation policy and procedures/processes. They are to be found in whichever care setting, hospital, home, community, residential home you may be working. The core care values should be promoted and are a sign of good practice.

Activity 1.4

If you are working in a care setting, check where your policy file is kept and identify if any information is held regarding the previously mentioned legislation. If you have access to the internet you can look up and obtain information about these laws.

Therefore, clients' rights are underpinned by underlying core care values and care is concerned with the welfare of clients including their rights as individuals. The final point to note is the issue of carers' rights which organisations should ensure are respected and the responsibility of clients not to be abusive or violent towards the carer.

Delivery of care

Currently in the UK, the ageing population is increasing. Many older people are fit and active but at some point it is likely that they will require health care. The development of guidelines regarding the safe delivery of care are therefore crucial. This section of the chapter sets the scene regarding the framework in which care delivery should operate as well as portraying the values upon which it should be based.

Care work means taking personal responsibility for one's own actions[21] as well as being sensitive to the consequences of our actions towards others. An individual should ensure that they have enough skill and knowledge to do the job, as for example, when moving and handling a client. Knowledge regarding health and safety at work and safe moving techniques/skills is vital. This is an area of dual responsibility, as employers should ensure that adequate training is available to acquire these skills. A carer needs to be aware of the boundaries and limitations of their role and how not to overstep such boundaries in order not to endanger the safety of the client or themselves.

Carers are often in a powerful position in relation to the person they are caring for because they are undertaking those activities which the client would normally do for themselves if they were able. Therefore the carer should always try to address this by making the client feel an equal partner. It is important to maintain client independence and choice at all times. In order to do this the carer must be mindful that individuals are ethnocentric, that is they have beliefs about health, religion, lifestyle and what they perceive to be right or wrong. Self-knowledge is important for carers for awareness of one's own health, beliefs and biases will make it easier to put them to one side when caring for someone else. It is crucial not to let bias, prejudice and stereotyping interfere with the quality of care we give to someone. To be empathetic, we must put our own thoughts and feelings to one side and try to see things totally from the client's point of view. In other words try to project yourself into seeing situations from the other person's perspective – as if you have had their life experience and education.

This can be difficult if we find that we hold different values. It may require considerable practice to think from the other person's point of view.

There may be occasions when the carer is unable to function in this way, for example, the carer may have been recently bereaved or is unable to be ethically sensitive, for instance regarding abortion. It may then be necessary for the carer to opt out of delivering care to that person. It is crucial that the carer recognises such a situation, is honest and speaks to someone about the dilemma. In an organisation, the manager or a senior colleague will be the person to approach.

The carer has a responsibility to take on the role of advocate, helping clients to achieve their goals and supporting their rights. Poor practice/standards should be challenged, as should stereotyping and prejudice, and any abuse witnessed or suspected should be reported immediately.

Activity 1.5

How would you describe good care? List the essential core care values you would include. Think about the kind of care you would like to receive if you were ill and being looked after by someone else.

NB: You can undertake this activity on your own and then check with someone else or do the activity in a group.

Although answers may differ, most people would suggest that care delivered should contain some of the following aspects:

- Dignity, respect of person
- To be treated equally
- Equal access to care resources
- Informed consent and the right to refuse treatment and care
- Advocacy on behalf of those who cannot speak for themselves
- To maintain, whenever possible, client independence and choice
- Trust and confidentiality

Respect of person

A person has the right to be treated with respect, dignity and as an individual and thus is entitled to an individual care plan. Health care legislation recognises that people are different and recommends that diversity should be embraced and that all clients should be treated fairly using anti-discriminatory practices. If a client complains, carers should know how to help them use procedures to register that complaint. All complaints should be investigated as soon as possible. In the past an overprotective or paternalistic approach was commonly undertaken and from the perspective of protecting vulnerable adults and children, decisions were made on behalf of the client. This should be avoided and the individual should be included in the decision-making process.

Developing anti-discriminatory practice

If practice shows disrespect and an intolerance of other groups, the behaviour and actions of the carer would indicate discriminatory practice. Everyone should be working to eradicate this type of approach and individuals/carers who demonstrate this type of behaviour should be challenged, especially if the client is being treated in a less favourable way and is disadvantaged by the carer's action. Certain groups are especially seen to be at risk of abuse: younger and older people, individuals with different sexual orientation, persons with disabilities, especially those with physical or hearing impairments, or those with learning difficulties or mental health problems.

The grouping together of individuals is known as stereotyping and can be labelling; again this should be challenged. Behaviour may include showing disrespect, name calling, making jokes, rationing care (even neglect) and/or perceiving clients as a burden.

Carers have the responsibility that no harm should come to the clients within their care. Abuse can be physical, sexual, psychological or financial and can also take the form of neglect or abandonment. Carers need to be vigilant to detect abuse and if suspected this information must be shared with the team, person in charge or GP; this information should be reported as soon as abuse is suspected. It is important to make a detailed written statement or complete an incident form and to make an entry in the individual's care plan.

Activity 1.6

Can you think of examples in practice that might lead to discrimination of certain individuals or groups? What effect might this have on the client? If recognised as an issue, how could it be discussed with colleagues? Could it be challenged? In what ways might the situation be improved?

There is legislation to protect clients. Think back to the legislation outlined earlier. It could cover the following:

- Equal opportunities
- The Race Relations Act 1976
- The Disability Discrimination Act 1995
- The Human Rights Act 1998

Once the move to eradicate anti-discriminatory practice has been made, the other concern is that the carer should consciously enter into a partnership with the client, incorporating the following:

- Respect of person and recognition of their physical, psychological and social needs
- To ensure privacy and dignity and give a duty of care to the individual
- Maintain independence and choice in care decisions

- Clients should retain control of their daily care and their activities of daily living and the carer should only step in if the person cannot do these things
- The carer should demonstrate empathy, show respect for the client and maintain the individual's self-esteem.

Informed consent

Prior to providing care to a client, their consent must be obtained. This is undertaken prior to a clinical procedure such as taking a temperature or blood pressure or a care activity, such as washing the client or taking them to the toilet. It is undertaken by approaching the client and greeting them, giving an explanation of your intentions and asking their permission to proceed; when the client responds the activity is undertaken. This process should be carried out on each occasion, even if the client is drowsy or unconscious. A formal consent in writing is obtained for invasive procedures, investigations and prior to surgery.

Advocacy

Whenever the delivery of care is embarked upon it should be realised that the carer has taken on the 'duty of care' on behalf of the client. The carer will thus act on that person's behalf, taking on the role of advocate for that person, supporting them and speaking out on their behalf, especially if they are unable to do so themselves.

Independence and choice

Although the carer delivers care and assumes the role of advocate for the client, the individual should always be able to retain their independence and have a choice in all situations, such as choosing foods from the menu or cleaning their own teeth. There may be times when someone is too ill and then the carer will intervene to take on the activities of daily living (e.g. washing, feeding) but once that person is able to do the activity for her- or himself, the carer will relinquish the activity back to the individual.

Trust and confidentiality

When someone else is caring for you it means that your privacy has been invaded by that person. As an adult you have carried out certain activities for yourself, e.g. washing, going to the toilet, feeding, moving around at will for many years. When you are ill or have a disability someone else may need to take over these activities for you, and for the client it can be demeaning, embarrassing and make them feel out of control of the situation. Linked to these activities of daily living is the disclosure to another person of much personal information. This information may not have been known to anyone else or only to those very close to that person. As a carer you have access to this knowledge and the client has put much trust into this relationship with you (the carer) and this must be respected at all times.

Confidentiality

Clients' rights are also incorporated into the issue of confidentiality of individuals' personal information. People divulge much personal information; in exchange, carers have a responsibility to honour this trust and keep the information confidential. It would only be shared with other members of the care team and disclosure is not even extended to the client's relatives or friends. Team members share the same information and this contributes to the quality of care delivered. Information about the client is written and documented in the client's care plan; these records should be written in clear handwriting or on a word procesor and must be accurate. Confidentiality and storage of information comes under the Data Protection Act and this topic is dealt with in more detail in Chapter 6. Informed consent, rights, responsibility and accountability are discussed from an ethical perspective in Chapter 2.

Universal precautions

A significant aspect of care in the early part of the twenty-first century is and will be to prevent and control infection. As clients' safety is still such a vital aspect of care the carer has a responsibility to obtain the relevant knowledge to do the job. In the early 1900s the commonest cause of death in the UK was infection. Today we are seeing the re-emergence of infection caused by bacteria resistant to the antibiotics in use and new or developing strains of viruses. Carers can do much to prevent cross-infection amongst clients. Universal precautions must be exercised in any risk situation; if working within an organisation the carer should refer to the unit/organisational policy/protocol. This will include correct handwashing, wearing protective clothing, use of plastic aprons and gloves, and the safe disposal of biological hazardous waste, linen and equipment. A more detailed discussion of this aspect of care is given in Chapter 9.

Legal restrictions

On occasion, legal restrictions operate in care, i.e. when individuals are non-competent by reason of confusion or have mental health problems or learning difficulties. It should be remembered that the nursing care action taken should be within the requirement of the law and the following are examples of legislation and regulations which need to be incorporated into the client's care plan.

- Mental health legislation
- Appointment of a legal guardian
- A court protection order
- Allocation of an enduring power of attorney
- Criminal convictions and immigration law

NB: minors under 18 years of age are under the jurisdiction of the law.

To protect the clients' rights all carers should understand the concepts regarding the standard/quality of care, and ensure that they work within the framework of legislation, policy and procedure.

> **Activity 1.7**
>
> When, where, and how would you raise issues and concerns regarding the standard of care? To whom would you go to register your concern?
>   There is no one right answer because it depends on the situation in which care is given, except to say disclosure may be in the public interest.

Usually the carer would voice his or her concern to the qualified nurse or the manager. There is no one right answer and the Public Disclosure Act 1998 supports carers who need to speak out.

Summary

Out of the core care values and human rights, certain principles of care have emerged which are seen as evidence of good care practice. As carers we should be consciously trying to incorporate these into all care work practices. Respect of persons and their families including those significant to them should be maintained. The preservation of clients' rights and dignity should underline all delivery of care.

In the UK, recognition and welcoming of diversity of clients in our multicultural society should be reflected in anti-discriminatory care practice and listening to the views of others and respecting them is of great importance. Confidentiality of all information held is sacrosanct and it is important that accurate well-written documentation is updated and held securely. It is also recognised that if individuals feel there has been an infringement they have the right to complain and should be given the necessary information to do so and carers should support individuals to access the complaints system. Finally, it is also important that the carer is protected and receives similar treatment by the employer.

References

1. Mann, J.M., Gruskin, S., Grodin, M.A. and Annas, G.J. (1999) *Human Rights: A reader*. Routledge, London.
2. United Nations (1948) *Universal Declaration of Human Rights*. United Nations, Geneva.
3. United Nations (1971) *Declaration on Rights of Mentally Retarded Persons*. United Nations, Geneva.
4. Department of Health (1974) *Health and Safety at Work Act 1974*. HMSO, London.
5. Home Office (1975) *Sex Discrimination Act 1975*. HMSO, London.
6. Home Office (1976) *Race Relations Discrimination Act 1976*. HMSO, London.
7. Department of Health (1982) *Mental Health (Amendment) Act 1982*. HMSO, London.
8. Department of Health (1983) *Mental Health Act 1983*. HMSO, London.
9. Department of Health (1986) *Disabled Persons Act 1986*. HMSO, London.

10. Department of Health (1989) *Children Act 1989*. HMSO, London.
11. Department of Health (1989) *Working Together Under the Children Act 1989*. HMSO, London.
12. Department of Health (1990) *National Health Service and Community Care Act 1990*. HMSO, London.
13. Department of Health (1990) *Food Safety Act 1990*. HMSO, London.
14. Department for Education and Employment (1995) *Disability Discrimination Act 1995*. HMSO, London.
15. Department of Health (1998) *Data Protection Act 1998*. HMSO, London.
16. Department of Health (1998) *Public Interest Disclosure Act 1998*. HMSO, London.
17. Department of Health (1998) *Human Rights Act 1998*. HMSO, London.
18. Department of Health (2000) *Care Standards Act 2000*. HMSO, London.
19. Department of Health (1991) *Patient's Charter 1991*. HMSO, London.
20. Department of Health (1995) *The Patient's Charter and You*. HMSO, London.
21. Royal College of Nursing (2004) *RCN Guidance on Professional Matter for Health Care Assistants and Nurse Cadets*. Royal College of Nursing, London.

Further reading

Baly, M. (1995) *Nursing and Social Change*, 3rd edn. Routledge, New York.
Department of Health (2002) *The Essence of Care: Client Focussed Benchmarking for Health Care Practitioners*. HMSO, London.
Gunn, C. (2001) *A Practical Guide to Complaint Handling*. Churchill Livingstone, Edinburgh.
Halloran, E.J. (ed.) (1995) *A Virginia Henderson Reader: Excellence in Nursing*. Springer, Berlin.
Henderson, V. (1966) *The Nature of Nursing*. Macmillan, New York.
Lang, M. (ed.) *Welfare Needs, Rights and Risks*. Routledge, London, in association with the Open University.
Roper, N., Logan, W. and Tierney, A.J. (2000) *The Roper, Logan, Tierney Model of Nursing: Based on the Activities of Daily Living*. Churchill Livingstone, Edinburgh.
Seedhouse, D. (1998) *Ethics: The Heart of Health Care*, 2nd edn. John Wiley and Sons, Hoboken, USA.
Thompson, I., Melia, K.M. and Boy, K.M. (2000) *Nursing Ethics*, 4th edn. Churchill Livingstone, Edinburgh.
Wilkinson, R. and Caulfield, H. (2000) *The Human Rights Act: A Practical Guide for Nurses*. Whurr Publishers, Biggleswade, UK.

Useful websites

European Court of Human Rights. www.dhdirhr.coe.fr (accessed February/March 2004).
Health Service Ombudsman Website. www.ombudsman.org.uk (accessed February/March 2004).
University of Minnesota Human Rights Library. www.umn.edu/humanrts (accessed February/March 2004).

Chapter 2
Ethics

Sandra Fortuna

Overview

This chapter aims to encourage the reader to think about ethical considerations in day-to-day life and in the work situation. It provides the opportunity to think about one's own ethics and the influence of the environment on one's ability to behave ethically. It highlights several dilemmas resulting from the application of ethical values to one's attitudes and behaviour in care situations. The chapter starts with a definition of ethics and its links with the law and human rights. It then follows the importance of ethics in care professions and the factors that impact on ethical decision making. Finally, it looks at specific dilemmas in ethical decision making in the work place.

Key words: Ethical values/principles; rights; human relationships; rules of behaviour; codes of conduct; policies; responsibilities; accountability; confidentiality; informed consent; choice; ethnic and cultural issues

Definition of ethics

Ethics can be described as a set of moral values/principles, which guide us in our actions and in making decisions in our day-to-day life. This ethic becomes enshrined in law, which in turn is applied in practice through codes of conduct and organisational policy. The codes of conduct and organisational policies are sets of rules that govern our behaviour in our relationships with others at work (including service users) in order to uphold such values. Examples of these values are: dignity, prudence, equality, honesty, openness and goodwill. Although these apply to all circumstances in our life and therefore to all professions, their expression varies according to:

1. The need of each profession for specific rules, e.g. in nursing professions the code of conduct includes rules for physical contact with clients when providing personal care. This does not apply in the same way to professions like psychology where physical contact is restricted.

2. The emphasis that each profession places on assuring that different rules are followed, e.g. psychotherapists may place greater emphasis on confidentiality rules than other professions.
3. The emphasis that the organisation places on different values, e.g. if the organisation emphasises the value of choice, it is likely that its policy to ensure this is more developed.

The basic ethical values mentioned in this chapter are stated in the United Nations *Universal Declaration of Human Rights*[1].

Activity 2.1

As an exercise to aid the thinking about ethics, it would be useful to list basic human rights that you value.

The list may include the following from the *Universal Declaration of Human Rights*[1]:

- Right to freedom and equality
- Right to dignity
- Right to life, liberty and security of person
- Right to freedom of opinion, thought and expression
- Right to privacy and respect
- Right to get married and have a family
- Right to education
- Right to own property

The human rights find expression in legal documents such as:

- Human Rights Act 1998
- Children Act 1989
- Health and Social Care Act 2001
- National Health Service and Community Care Act 1990
- Patient's Charter 1990
- Mental Health Act Code of Practice 1993
- Access to Health Records Act 1990
- Data Protection Act 1998

When applied in practice and expressed in codes and policies, these documents are subject to developments through time. These are influenced by increased professional knowledge and awareness of injustice and by the views of society in general.

Carers need to know the written policies in the workplace to be up to date with changes over time. If there is no written policy, carers need to be aware that moral values are being expressed in their behaviour and that of other professionals. It is thus important to think about these issues.

Activity 2.2

In this context, write a list of rules which could be included in a code of conduct for carers in order to follow the human rights and the values they embody.

When writing this list one may find that these rules do not provide fixed answers. They cannot cover all situations that one encounters in the workplace. Rather, they provide guidance towards different points that need considering, to enable one to reach decisions which are in the best interest of all concerned (i.e. the person, the carers, the family and the other service users he/she comes in contact with), in the light of the current knowledge.

There are situations where one cannot find a right answer that would be beneficial for all concerned even with the guidance of the ethical values/principles. These situations constitute dilemmas. An example of a dilemma is the situation where a client is refusing to eat and the treatment team needs to decide whether to respect the client's right of choice or to respect the value of preserving life and thus force-feed them.

Importance of ethics in the health and social care professions

Ethics in care professions are not only applicable to major decisions made by health or care management teams. They also apply to the minor daily decisions which a carer has to make on the spot. These decisions can be difficult and sometimes create dilemmas in which the carer cannot respect both the person's own rights and the rights of others around him or her. The dilemmas can lead to difficulties in keeping consistency of one's own decisions over time and of different team members' decisions in relation to the same service user, for example the situation where a carer has to decide between allowing the person to choose when to go to bed or follow the organisation's policy about bed time.

Observation of the rules based on ethical principles and the team's thinking that goes with such observation can give a sense of fairness and balance to difficult decisions. Take for example, the situation where a service user with learning disabilities is not consenting to have blood tests but is likely to have a life-threatening condition. Ethical codes enable the health team to think about which decision is likely to promote the best results for the service user whilst respecting the person's right to consent. Care assistants may be expected to participate in the multi-disciplinary team's decision as to whether the person has the capacity to give consent and whether the physical needs outweigh this right in any case. Without the rules and the team's collective observation of those, the service user could either be subjected to abuse of power (e.g. by the decision to sedate the person in order to give them the blood test), or negligence (e.g. by the decision not to give the person the test under the pretext of respecting their right to give consent with all the consequences this could bring).

In other words, as a carer it is important to know the law that embodies the ethical values in order to deal with the constant decisions which have to be made in the work environment. This knowledge helps the carer to make prompt ethical decisions, to protect the rights of the service users and to avoid situations where no decisions are made. Taking the previous example, if the ethical guidelines had not been in place, the team could be paralysed by anxiety. This could lead to serious consequences for the person and for themselves.

Personal and environmental influences in ethical decision-making

So far this chapter has been considering the ethical values that are set down in the work place from policies and codes of conduct. However, it is vital that one considers the internal/personal moral values that one brings to the workplace. In fact, our ethical behaviour takes these rules of our workplace into account, but is also dependent on our own good intentions and our own values learned during our formative years.

Difficulties can arise when there is a mismatch between intention and behaviour. A carer who follows sound policies 'because he or she is told to do so' but has different internal values, may be acting ethically and have an apparently satisfactory ethical attitude. However, another carer, whose internal values are in accordance with the ethical rules of the policies, is far more likely to achieve durable results in respecting the service user's rights and developing healthy relationships in the workplace. Another mismatch can occur when the organisation is felt by the carer to be at fault in respecting human rights, creating a situation in which it is impossible for the carer to remain in the job. Thus it is important to be aware of these possible mismatches and their consequences. One needs to be aware and question one's own moral values in order to avoid behaving in a manner which could hinder the service user's rights. For example, consider the following situation: A care assistant working in an elderly people's home follows the policy of asking the clients' permission to provide information to relatives about the care. However, this carer believes that this policy should not be implemented with older clients when the families have to pay for the care. How easy would it be for this carer to be consistent in following the rules?

Our emotions and prejudices affect our judgement and may lead to justifying one's actions as ethical when they are not. For example, one may be less inclined to take action if a person with learning disabilities steals than if an adolescent of average intelligence steals. One may see them as people who do not have the ability to commit crimes. One may justify one's reluctance to take action by saying: 'They can't help it', without further exploring why they are doing so. In this case we are depriving the service users of learning from the consequences of their actions.

When working in health and social care, it is important to be aware of environmental factors that may create difficulties in making ethical decisions. One difficulty can be to follow certain rules in an organisation where it may have become common through time to ignore them. Teams where these matters are discussed on a regular basis are more likely to develop cohesion and consistency in following ethical rules.

Work environments where stress is high, workloads too demanding and support structures (e.g. supervision) limited, create conditions where carers can overlook ethical issues. In such circumstances our ability to make decisions is likely to be clouded by the tendency to 'take short cuts'. Where staff feel overwhelmed and resentful decisions/actions are more likely to be affected by emotional states. Take, for example, a day centre for adults with mental health difficulties, which is very busy, short-staffed and a carer key-works several people. This carer knows the policy about respecting clients' privacy and confidentiality when obtaining information from them, but in such an environment how possible would it be to respect this policy? How could information be obtained from the client when there are inadequate space conditions? When and how could discussion of cases happen with professionals without their being overheard?

Another example of the influence of the environment in our decision-making is as follows: In a community trust where all workers have access to other workers' files a carer has a common case with another member of the team and needs information from a report. The secretary tells the carer that everyone photocopies reports from each other's files. How does the carer proceed? Does he or she consult the colleague in question or do they copy the report as everyone else does? What would they do if that person refuses to provide the information?

These are questions that may not have an immediate answer and flexibility is needed when thinking about circumstances involving the decision-making process. However, especially when difficulties arise in following ethical guidelines, it is important to bear these issues in mind to ensure that one considers *all* possibilities before making a judgement. It is this constant consideration and reflection that can contribute to the review of policy guidelines.

Ethical issues

As highlighted throughout this chapter, ethical values are not always easy to apply. This part of the chapter highlights some specific issues that one may come across in work as a care assistant and aims to increase awareness of their complexity in day-to-day decision making.

Confidentiality

Confidentiality protects the person's right to privacy and is a widely used term in health and social care settings. But what do we really mean by confidentiality? Different people may give different definitions. As an exercise it would be useful to ask two people working in different places what they understand by the term 'confidentiality'. It is possible to find that the definitions vary according to the settings they are working in, the group they work for and their personal views.

Confidentiality means that information given by or observed about service users should not be disclosed to anyone else without consent. For children and adults unable to give consent, this responsibility for consent is laid on the parents or legal guardian. However, there are situations when it is important that information is disclosed even without consent. A carer would not make decisions as to whether information should be disclosed on his or her own. A senior person should be available to discuss the issue with them. However, in the eventuality of not having access to a senior person when the situation arises, it is important for the carer to be aware of which situations demand disclosure:

- If it is in the public's best interests, e.g. if the service user indicates in any way that he or she is going to harm others, physically, sexually, emotionally
- If the court requests information (under certain circumstances)
- If it is in the person's best interests, e.g. if the person indicates that he or she is going to harm him- or herself or is at risk of being harmed.

Although these are the general rules, there are exceptions to the rules for other reasons. Confidentiality applies to information passed on verbally and in writing. It is important that the information recorded is accurate, clear and legible and that the records are kept in a safe place. This can create difficulties in keeping records. For example, the service user may say that they do not want the information written down. Again a decision will have to be made as to whether this is safe for the carer or the service user, e.g. in case of later allegation of neglect. The policies of the organisation for record keeping are of great importance in this decision.

Another aspect is to decide who should know about a particular piece of information. The Data Protection Act 1998[2] states that disclosure of information should be 'on a need to know basis' (see also Chapter 6). For example, in the case of disclosing information to a therapist working with the service user, it may be difficult to decide which information the therapist needs to know about the person in order to work as effectively as possible.

Although in both cases described above the situation needs to be discussed with senior staff before decisions are made, it is important as a carer to bear in mind:

- The rights to privacy, trust and respect of the service user
- The ability of the service user to give consent
- Whether disclosing information without the service user's consent is in their best interests
- Whether disclosing information without the service user's consent is going to damage your trust relationship with the person
- Whether withholding information is going to be detrimental for the service user (e.g. by causing a split in the approaches of different carers and professionals involved).

Informed consent and choice

Informed consent relates to the service user's right to make choices when provided with information about several possibilities. Carers need to make decisions on a day-to-day basis about the person's ability to consent in situations that are ordinary.

Activity 2.3

Write down the factors that a carer may have to consider when deciding whether a person can make choices.

The list may include:

- The person's ability to understand the effects of an activity, e.g. staying up late and not getting enough sleep and rest
- The effects that staying up may have on others around the person, e.g. is the person keeping others awake?
- The benefit of an activity on the person's development, e.g. is the person learning new skills or acquiring knowledge?

The ability to make choices and consent requires the person to be able to take into account *all* aspects of a decision. This becomes an issue particularly when working with groups where the ability to give consent and make choices is not clear. Examples of these groups are children, adults with learning disabilities, older adults suffering from dementia and adults with brain injuries.

When working with these groups one needs to be aware of the psychological and social factors influencing our judgement about whether to provide the choice to the person: our perceptions and expectations about the person's capacity to consent influence the amount of choice given. Society tends to see these groups as unable to make choices in their best interests. Take as an example the consent to intimate relationships. In working with an adult with learning disabilities who is seen as unable to understand the consequences of such relationships (i.e. pregnancy, sexually transmitted illness), one may feel compelled to dissuade the person from pursuing them. Alternatively, one could consider:

- Further education for the person about, e.g. physiological matters, sexually transmitted illnesses and contraception
- An assessment of the person's capacity to consent within a relationship.

Another aspect that may need consideration is the work with the person's family and social networks in understanding the issues of adhering to ethical values. The belief that the person is vulnerable if allowed the right to make the choice to have intimate relationships may prevent a carer from encouraging the person to live a fulfilling life. Allowing people to make choices involves taking risks but it also allows for personal development. In some cases carers may be asked to balance the risk in a way that does not jeopardise the reputation of the organisation they work for. Taking the previous example, in order to enable the service user to fulfil his or her potential, a carer would need to support the person to give consent to the best of their ability. In doing so, this carer could face opposition from his or her manager because if the person were to become involved in harmful relationships, the organisation could be seen as contributing to that situation.

A subtle aspect of helping a service user to make choices is the relationship between the carer and the person. Naturally, a carer will be seen in a position of power and being in this position, it is difficult not to influence the person's decision.

The capacity to give consent involves complex abilities such as the ability to consider different information; to relate the information to long-term consequences; to imagine the consequences and the feelings elicited by them; and to relate all these factors in making the decision. Thus it is important to deliver information in a manner the person can understand and to take time to explain and explore the different aspects. Service users may be able to make some decisions but not others. Therefore, there is the need to judge at any given moment which decisions can be made by the person, e.g. the person may be able to make decisions about which activity to pursue that day, but not be able to make an informed decision as to whether they want to go on holiday next year.

A carer will be faced with daily situations where he or she has to decide whether the person is competent to make choices and decisions about different aspects of their lives. A general rule is to maximise the person's competence and independence but not present impossible tasks.

Rights and responsibilities

Rights and responsibilities go hand in hand. The in-depth exploration of the different types of responsibility and rights of a carer is beyond the scope of this chapter. However, what is appropriate to raise here are the dilemmas related to the exercise of such responsibilities and rights. A care assistant has responsibility towards the service user, the family, the organisation, him- or herself and the wider society. When making ethical decisions it is not always easy to reconcile the rights of all these people and to decide where the responsibility rests.

For instance, the right to have intimate relationships is about responsibilities and rights. A carer's primary responsibility is to the service user. In this context, the primary responsibility would be to support the person to fulfil their sexual needs. However, this can involve risk taking and lead to complications for the organisation towards which the carer also has responsibility. This conflict is difficult to resolve and there is often need for multi-disciplinary decisions. This encourages shared responsibility for the risk and promotes a safer context in which to support the service user.

Care assistants are also faced with other dilemmas about the rights and the responsibilities towards service users. Take as an example a client with severe and enduring mental illness living in a continuing care unit, who refuses to eat. The person has the ability to consent but is putting their life at risk by not eating. As an exercise, it would be useful to think about what would prevail: the person's right to choose not to eat; or the responsibility of the carer to keep the person alive.

This is another dilemma, which does not have an easy answer. Again a decision by a multi-disciplinary team would be needed in order to act in the person's best interests on the basis of current knowledge and the law.

Sometimes it can be difficult to decide towards whom one has primary responsibility. This situation is common when working with children or dependent adults. In this case, although the service user is the child or the dependent adult, families need to have some information about the person. This may obscure the focus for the primary responsibility.

So far, this section has dealt with the rights of the service user and responsibilities of carers. However, it is important to highlight that carers also have rights and that the service users, their families, the organisation and the wider community need to respect those. The rights of a carer include statutory rights, the rights that the profession gives them within the boundaries of codes of conduct and personal rights similar to those of the service user (although these are often not written).

Carers working in social and health care have fundamental rights which are not always acknowledged: the right to further education, the right to supervision and the right of access to management for consultation.

Accountability

Accountability involves taking responsibility for one's actions. It is about being able to justify one's behaviour, by explaining the reasons behind any given decision, and being aware of the possible consequences which will result from it. This implies that one needs knowledge and understanding to make informed decisions and has the authority to act on them individually. A carer may face dilemmas related to different types of accountability. An example of this is if the carer makes a decision against the policy of the organisation, but one which is morally sound, e.g. when the policy states that clients should not smoke when in acute mental health hospitals, but the effects of not smoking are causing the client great distress.

Care assistants are direct carers and as such they are often faced with situations when they must make ethical decisions without the support of a senior worker or even may be pressured to make decisions that are beyond the limits of their knowledge and understanding. It is important that they become aware of which decisions are in the realm of their abilities and which decisions they need to consult about with a senior member of staff. It is here that accessibility to senior members of staff for consultation has an important role to play.

In this context, supervision provides a forum to think about one's attitudes and behaviours and to reflect upon one's rational for such behaviours. It also gives the opportunity to discuss different interpretations of rules.

Ethnic/cultural differences

This final section looks at some of the dilemmas carers may face when working with service users from another culture. Basic ethical values are universal. However, there are some that have cultural variations. This requires one to examine those variations and find ways to challenge one's preconceptions and moral ethics. For example, in some cultures the family, rather than the individual, is seen as a unit. This creates difficulties in, e.g. keeping confidentiality or enabling the person to exercise his or her rights to self-determination when the person's choices differs from those of his or her family.

Activity 2.4

A helpful exercise is to think about and make a list of which 'rules of thumb' a carer needs to follow in order to consider cultural differences when making ethical decisions.

The list may include some of those mentioned by Francis[3]:

- Ask rather than assert
- The *expression* of values may vary with culture although the values may be the same
- Be sensitive to costume unless there is a good reason not to be
- Respect touching taboos
- Be aware of greetings and forms of address

Summary

This chapter looked at the definition of ethics, its links with the law and its expression through codes of conduct and policy. It also explored different dilemmas that carers have to face, the importance of a reflective approach to their work (through the use of supervision) and the importance of consultation with senior staff or managers in making sound ethical decisions.

Acknowledgements

Thank you to Pat Bishop for the help in preparing this chapter and to Isabelle Mitchell and Frank Garvey for their feedback.

References

1. United Nations (1948) *Universal Declaration of Human Rights*. United Nations, Geneva.
2. Department of Health (1998) *Data Protection Act 1998*. HMSO, London.
3. Francis, R. (1999) *Ethics for Psychologists*. BPS Books, Leicester.

Further Reading

Department of Health (1989) *Children Act 1989*. HMSO, London.
Department of Health (1990) *Access to Health Records Act 1990*. HMSO, London.

Department of Health (1990) *National Health Service and Community Care Act*. HMSO, London.

Department of Health (1990; 1993) The *Patient's Charter* and the *Mental Health Act Code of Practice*. HMSO, London.

Department of Health (1998) *Data Protection Act 1998*. HMSO, London.

Department of Health (1998) *Human Rights Act 1998*. HMSO, London.

Department of Health (2001) *Health and Social Care Act 2001*. HMSO, London.

Tschudin, V. (1993) *Ethics: Nurses and Patients*. Scutari Press, London.

Chapter 3
Individuality and diversity

Hazel Heath and Lynne Phair

Overview

Each person is unique. Human beings are born of different races, ethnicities and religions, with wide-ranging abilities, into vastly different circumstances. People's lives encompass the broadest spectrum of experiences and, as a result of each of these unique combinations, individual beliefs, values and attitudes develop. Every human being is therefore an expression of infinite individuality.

In caring work it is fundamental that we appreciate the uniqueness of every individual with whom we work, but this is not always easy to achieve, particularly with people who are very different from ourselves or have led very different lives. For example, it can be difficult for young people to understand the life experiences and perspectives of someone who has lived for 80 years, or for someone living in a European town to understand life in an African village. Lack of understanding of the individuality of others and the range of diversity within the communities we live in can lead to prejudice and discrimination. The effects of this in health and social care can be particularly devastating because service users are mostly vulnerable in some way.

This chapter broadly explains some elements of individuality and identity, including gender, race, ethnicity and culture, life experiences and life circumstances, abilities and disabilities, health and illness, and sexuality. Then issues underpinning how we work with individuality and diversity are explored, including rights, responsibilities, prejudice and discrimination. The chapter concludes with a discussion of essential issues in care such as supporting individual rights. In order to balance the content of this chapter with the remainder of the book, the topic of sexuality is discussed in more detail than other aspects of individuality and diversity. Throughout the chapter the key concepts are illustrated with examples from a range of settings, which we have called 'Practice to Care'.

It is important to emphasise that, while elements of individuality are considered under headings, these should not be used to 'label' people. Within any category, people vary greatly, and should be viewed and treated as unique individuals. To quote Coleen Wedderburn Tate[1]: 'Diversity is not an add-on. Ultimately it is beyond religion, gender, sexual orientation, disability . . . beyond the visible'.

Key words: Individual; gender; identity; sexuality; race; culture; religion; ethnicity; diversity; attitudes; beliefs; values; life experience; abilities/disabilities; health/ill health

Individuality and individual identity

Gender

Gender denotes male or female. It may be identified biologically, in terms of roles or in terms of one's identity.

Biological gender

Whether we are born as male or female is determined by the chromosomes we acquire at the moment of conception and full development of gender characteristics takes place during puberty when the secondary sexual characteristics come to fruition as a result of hormone changes. Females develop a curvy body shape, breasts and start to menstruate. Males develop more body muscle and body hair and their voices deepen. The penis and testicles enlarge. Once puberty is complete both males and females are capable of producing children themselves.

Gender roles

Within most cultures and some religions males and females have traditionally had different roles, for example men as breadwinners, women in home-making and child-rearing, although of course many individuals choose not to live according to these traditions.

Gender identity

Gender identity means whether we identify ourselves as male or female. For some people gender identity is straightforward, e.g. a person born with a male body identifies himself as a male and is happy to live within the prescribed traditions of his culture as a male. For others, gender identity is less straightforward, for example a person is biologically male but identifies as a female. Such persons can experience enormous distress as, although they are viewed and treated as male, this denies how they really want to be and how they are as a person – a female. Some individuals may be uncertain about their gender identity and may wish to be identified sometimes as a male and sometimes as a female. Others may not want to be assigned a gender identity at all but just be accepted as the individuals they feel themselves to be inside. Some individuals change their biological gender to match their gender identity.

Practice to care

Understanding of gender issues affects how care workers approach and respond to clients and thus the care they give. Using this knowledge in a practical way will assist us to ensure that we do not make assumptions about aspects of a person's life.

Gender issues are very relevant when considering the role of informal carers. It is often assumed that the woman in a relationship will take on the caring role, or that she will not need to be offered a home-help service to do the shopping or cooking because she will know how to do this. Equally women who become carers are rarely offered lessons in how to manage what may be perceived as 'the work of the man in the home'; tasks such as checking the oil in the car or mowing the lawn.

Within a care setting gender issues can be managed better if staff think to offer clients the night clothes they want to wear rather than assuming men will want pyjamas and women a nightgown. In order to prevent their attitudes communicating through their facial expression or actions, care staff must be conscious of their own feelings towards, for example, a man who wishes to dress as a woman. By coming to terms with their own feelings, rather than demonstrating shock or lack of understanding, care workers will be better able to support clients at their time of need.

Race, ethnicity, culture and religion

Race

The term race can be defined differently. Assumptions of race can be made on the basis of superficial biological differences such as skin colour, bone structure or hair type. Race can identify where people were born, e.g. Irish, or describe how they identify their origins, e.g. African American or Asian British.

Ethnicity

Ethnicity indicates identification with a common homeland, shared history, common language or dialect, religion or a distinctive culture.

Culture

A less broad term than ethnicity, culture is variously defined but generally refers to a distinctive way of life that encompasses common understandings learned and shared within a group. Cultural beliefs and values guide behaviour in terms of accepted norms, values and behaviours within a community and there are dynamic aspects of culture that pass on through generations or change over time. Culture influences individuals in powerful subconscious ways and food is strongly associated with culture. Culture is not something unique to people who have a non-British ethnic background. Every region, every area of the country, and sometimes even a village or town may have some specific cultural aspect in their way of life that will cause distress if it is not carried out. People from a mining town may have a very different approach to life than people who live in a rural village; different festivals may be celebrated in different ways and different foods may be relevant.

Religion

Religion pertains to beliefs, values and codes of behaviour which are fundamental to many people's lives.

Practice to care

As the UK becomes more multi-cultural it is vital that care workers understand
that different religions, cultures and ethnic backgrounds will profoundly influence the care a person wants. There are too many different aspects to be able to
list them all and individuals, even within the same group, will vary considerably, but the ward, domiciliary office or care home should have a reference book
to ensure that staff can read about any specific customs and practices that a
person may wish to uphold.

Some faiths have rituals in relation to using the toilet. For example, for people
whose cultural practice is to use their right hand to cleanse themselves after
using the toilet, a jug may need to be placed in the toilet or the position of
handrails assessed. People from some religions, e.g. Islam, may wish to pray
during the day. In this case we must work with clients to establish how this can
be achieved and their care needs met. Talking to individual persons and asking
them how they want to be helped is vital. If a care worker has to stay to support
the patient during religious practices, total respect must be shown.

In care home settings where celebration of festivals is popular, the racial, ethnic
and religious customs of every resident should be respected and the festivals of
all of the residents should be considered.

The key to giving positive care regarding people's race and ethnicity is to talk
to them, and ask how they can be helped to uphold their beliefs. Individuals may
not want to practise the traditional customs of their particular culture or religion
and assuming participation is as damaging to the person's self-esteem and rights,
as not ensuring participation if this is desired.

Life circumstances and life experiences

Advantage/disadvantage

The circumstances into which people are born strongly influence their lifestyles,
health and even how long they live. People living in polluted areas with poor
quality housing and inadequate food generally have shorter lifespans than those
living in non-polluted areas with good housing and nutrition. People can also
be advantaged or disadvantaged in terms of life circumstances and opportunities. A person born into a loving and secure family unit, who is supported
through their development, receives a sound education and earns a high income
will have greater resources to draw upon in times of trouble or illness than
someone who does not have these advantages. Such advantages or disadvantages, of course, in no way affect the value of individuals as human beings, their
abilities or what they have to offer in life.

Life experiences

Age merely denotes the number of years we have lived. It does not indicate what we are like as people. Attitudes to old and young can be negative, with older people viewed as out of date or not worth the effort and younger people being viewed as rebellious or disruptive. Neither stereotype is true and, in fact, the only factor distinguishing older people from younger people is that they have lived longer and lived through different times. Very old people have seen massive changes from writing with chalk on slate to the World Wide Web and from horse-drawn carriages to space travel. Wisdom can be gained through life experiences and in many cultures the elders are valued as the custodians of cultural wisdom.

Practice to care

Life experiences will affect the way a person wants to be cared for and sometimes how they expect to be cared for, but they must never become a basis on which care workers decide the level of respect they show. This would be discrimination. We should never make assumptions that because someone has experienced deprivation they do not need the best care because they 'won't know any different' or that because a client is known to be affluent that he or she has a right to expect preferential treatment. The standard of care, the respect shown to clients and residents and the way they are spoken to must be the same for everyone.

Life experiences will affect how clients respond to care and from whom they can accept care. This is particularly relevant for someone who has cognitive impairment or dementia. This person may not understand what is happening, or may mistake a care worker for someone they knew in their past. This may be positive but it could be negative, especially if they have experienced trauma, perhaps during a war. Care workers should talk to the families to ascertain if there are any life experiences that could affect the person's acceptance of care or certain staff members.

Other aspects of lifestyle and experience may affect how someone accepts the routine of care. Perhaps someone has had a dirty job and always bathed at night, or only shaved on a Sunday, or only changed their socks on a Tuesday and Friday for their own personal reasons. These aspects of care may seem small but, if not upheld, can cause resentment in patients who feel that their individuality is being taken away while the institution's rituals are being forced upon them. If there are no real care-related reasons why individual preference of lifestyle is not upheld, the removal of such rights and choices could be considered abusive.

The important factor is to talk with the client and family, find out what aspects of their lifestyle are important to them and, without making any judgements, uphold these as far as possible.

Abilities and disabilities

Each individual has a range of abilities and disabilities, and disability in one aspect of life does not preclude achievement in others, for example well-known individuals such as Professor Stephen Hawking who, with the assistance of tech-nology has achieved renowned scientific discoveries, Tanni Grey-Thompson who, with the aid of a wheelchair, has achieved sporting prowess, and the Chicken Shed Theatre company in which children of all abilities perform acclaimed theatrical productions.

The diversity of causes and effects of disability is immense and each person's experience is unique, yet there is a tendency to lump people together, for example wheelchair users, and label them as 'the disabled'. Just because someone has different physical or mental abilities from others does not mean that he or she is disabled.

People may be disabled by visual or hearing impairment, pain, fatigue, the effects of chronic illness such as Parkinson's disease or a part of the body not functioning. Many people with disabilities experience disadvantage in life, such as low income, isolation and lack of access to communities or services.

Practice to care

The most important factor in care workers applying knowledge about ability and disability is not automatically doing something just because someone looks as if they might not be able to do it for themselves. When a person with a disability arrives in any care setting, care workers should ask how they can best assist him or her, or indeed if there is anything with which they would like help. It may be that the person just needs things positioned in a certain place, or needs time to complete personal tasks. Individuals may have special equipment to assist them. In this case care workers should obtain permission to place identification on it and record how staff are to assist with its use.

People who live with a disability know what they can and cannot do, and they are the experts. Each person develops his or her individual ways of living life, and staff must respect that. The golden rule is that every person is independent unless he or she says, or staff observe, that they are unable to manage.

Health and ill-health

Although most people retain reasonable health throughout their lives, individ-uals can be born with ill-health or this can develop at any stage. Health is affected by many factors such as our environment, the air we breathe, what we eat and the quality of housing we inhabit. It is also affected by lifestyle in terms of whether we smoke, exercise sufficiently or take harmful substances in excess. Certain diseases are linked to particular geographical areas, cultural groups or socio-economic circumstances, and the link between poverty and ill-health has frequently been made.

When ill-health seemingly arises through lifestyle there can be blame, for example a significant number of middle-aged and older people have breathing problems due to smoking or exposure to environmental pollutants. When they were younger, however, there was little understanding about the dangers of smoking, asbestos or radiation. Another example could be the high incidence of pregnancy and sexually transmitted infections in certain parts of the world. If understanding about contraception or safer sexual practices has not reached them, they have less control over their conditions. The incidence of drug and alcohol misuse is increasing, and its effects on health are well documented, but people in this situation need understanding and help rather than condemnation.

Some illnesses attract prejudice or stigma, for example mental illness, sexually transmitted infections and human immunodeficiency virus/acquired immune deficiency syndrome (HIV/AIDS). Sometimes these diseases are associated with practices which are traditionally morally condemned or the least well understood, so the stigma is to some extent based on the fear of the unknown.

Practice to care

Understanding and accepting that clients' ill-health has been caused by their lifestyles, someone else's lifestyle or the circumstances in which they have lived, can enable us to manage our own views or prejudices about why the person has decided to live that way. As always, however, it is dangerous to make assumptions. Clients may not wish to discuss how they became ill and, although the illness may be thought to have been self-induced, this may not be the case. A famous example is the entertainer Roy Castle who died with lung cancer yet had never smoked. He suffered because, as he worked, he inhaled the smoke in the clubs where he performed (passive smoking).

The role of the care worker is to care for the person in whatever way they wish, in whatever way is needed. Health and social care professionals will identify whether the person's lifestyle has caused the ill-health and will work with him or her to address this.

Caring for a person who suffers ill-health because of lifestyle should be no different from caring for any other person. The care worker should report any observations or information that may be helpful to the professionals working with individual persons to improve their health. Clients may speak to care workers about problems and, while not disclosing this information to anyone other than the relevant professional, and with the agreement (or knowledge if the information is very serious) of the individual, care workers should pass on information to help in promoting the client's health. For example, someone may disclose that a partner is abusing them, or that their finances are so bad they cannot afford appropriate food or medicines. This type of information can be dealt with, with the client's permission, and subsequently their health can be improved. Care workers should not withhold information (see Chapter 2 for details about confidentiality), as they may not have the knowledge or the accountability to best judge its relevance to that person's health and possible recovery.

Sexuality

Sexuality is an important, but often challenging and neglected, area of care for professionals and care workers alike. Broadly, sexuality encompasses how we see ourselves, how we identify ourselves and whom we choose for love and intimacy. It is expressed through our thoughts and behaviours, personal presentation, sensuality, relationships and roles in life.

Specifically sexuality[2]:

- Is an essential integrated element of the whole person
- Is a creative force in human experience
- Is a fundamental aspect of how individuals relate to one another
- Embraces personal choice and tolerance of difference

Sexuality encompasses:

- Self-concept, sexual identity and sexual orientation
- Psychological, social, cultural, spiritual and biological elements

Sexuality is expressed:

- By human beings in health, illness and disability
- Throughout the lifespan
- Through personal thoughts, feelings, behaviours, presentation, sensuality, intimacy and roles in life
- Negatively through power dynamics such as in rape, sexual abuse and sexual harassment

A more narrow idea of sexuality is commonly used. This focuses on sexual preference, that is, to whom we are attracted and with whom we seek intimate relationships. 'Heterosexuality' indicates attraction to a different gender, i.e. male to female and vice versa. 'Homosexuality' (pronounced as in 'hot') indicates an attraction to one's own gender. Correctly used, the term 'homosexual' (pronounced as in 'home') indicates males sexually attracted to males. 'Bisexual' indicates that individuals are attracted to both males and females.

Challenges

Working with sexuality in care, or even acknowledging it, is challenging because:

- Anything to do with sex can be embarrassing
- It can be difficult to contemplate some people 'having sex'
- We all bring our own individual identities, experiences and 'sexualities'

Sexual imagery and references to sex are all around us in our everyday lives yet, despite this, it can be embarrassing for us to consider, address and discuss sex, sexuality or sexual health, even with those closest to us. In care settings we become very accustomed to asking our clients 'How are your bowels?', but asking them about sex-related matters can seem so much more embarrassing.

We can also find it difficult, sometimes impossible, to contemplate some other people as sexual beings, as wanting to express themselves sexually and to 'have sex'. This is particularly so for groups such as:

- Our parents, grandparents and older people generally
- Children
- People with disabilities, both physical and in learning

- People who are disfigured
- People affected by sexually transmitted infections, including HIV and AIDS
- People who are dying and particularly those close to death

There is no factual basis to such perceptions in that there is no reason why these people should desire a sexual identity any less than everyone else.

We all bring our own 'sexualities', sexual identities and experiences into the care situation. For example we may be in or out of love, celibate or sexually active, hetero-, homo- or bisexual and, within each of these categories, we may be happily fulfilled or experiencing difficulties.

Partly due to these challenges, sexuality is commonly neglected in care. With the exception of services focusing on the genital organs and their functioning, such as gynaecology or genitourinary medicine, on reproduction, such as midwifery, or those specifically promoting sexual health, sexuality is largely neglected because of some common misconceptions. Reasons for its neglect include:

- Sexuality is not considered a priority when people are ill or in need of care.
- Sexuality often does not seem obviously relevant in the current care situation.
- We do not always understand much about sexuality.

A common misconception in most care settings is that sexuality is unimportant. We might question how it can be a priority for people who are, for example, acutely ill (such as with a heart attack or stroke), have chronic illness (such as chronic pulmonary disease, diabetes mellitus, Parkinson's disease or cancer), or who are dying. Yet, at such difficult times, what could be more natural than wanting to be close to those we love. Affectionate and intimate relationships can be highly comforting and supportive to people who are ill.

How health influences sexuality may not be obvious, particularly in such conditions as pain, breathlessness, incontinence, limited joint mobility or when taking certain medicines. In addition, and particularly with some client groups, there is insufficient knowledge for evidence-based care and about which we understand little such as minority ethnic groups and lesbians, homosexuals, bisexuals or transsexuals.

Working constructively with sexuality in care

In care settings, professional priorities and care regimens often assume greater importance than a client's desire for self-expression or intimate relationships, for example a person with chronic pain or disability living at home may find the best time for intimacy with a partner is during the afternoon but that this is not possible because the community care team want to deliver personal care at this time.

Preserving a person's intimate relationships is very important. Often, particularly for people who are older, chronically ill or disabled, once intimate relationships are interrupted, for example through hospital admission, they never resume.

It is important to create an environment that acknowledges sexuality as part of the care agenda and challenges inappropriate barriers to its expression. For example:

- The layout of the environment should afford privacy for conversations and for couples to be together undisturbed.
- Information leaflets should be available, for example on sex after a stroke, advice services for people with disabilities, or sexually transmitted infections. Information should be available in a range of formats (e.g. large print or audiotape) and represent the range of clients using the service, including those from minority ethnic groups and those who are lesbian or homosexual.
- Clients should be asked if they are happy to receive care from someone of the opposite gender.
- Clients should be able to choose when services are delivered, particularly at home.

Research shows that clients prefer issues related to sexuality to be raised by health professionals but care workers often come across these issues. It is important to work within your own competence in terms of your knowledge and skills and to refer to someone with greater expertise when necessary.

It is also important to recognise that sexuality might not be relevant to a person's care or, even if it is, the individual can choose not to disclose information. Individual choice in this matter must be respected.

Diversity among individuals

The topics discussed so far are merely broad categories, which can serve to identify individuals or groups of people. It is important to recognise, however, that within each category every person is distinct and the potential for diversity is thus infinite.

The elements discussed above not only distinguish us as individuals, they strongly influence our beliefs, values and attitudes (Fig. 3.1). These are important to identify in our work with other people.

Working with individuality and diversity

Attitudes, beliefs, values

Our beliefs, values and attitudes influence how we perceive others and how we work with them. Although these are deeply held they can change and when our beliefs, attitudes or values negatively influence how we care for others, they must be identified and challenged.

Beliefs

These are ideas, principles or propositions that we accept as true. They are often based more on faith than fact, for example the belief that most people are basically nice.

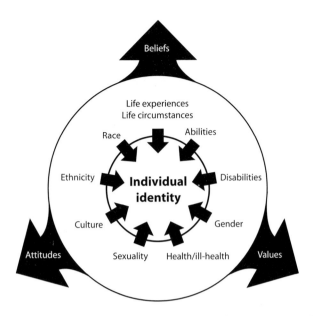

Fig. 3.1 The influence of elements of individuality on beliefs, values and attitudes.

Attitude

Attitudes can be seen in the ways in which we view something or someone. They often imply some judgement and manifest in the way we treat others. For example if we believe that most people are basically nice, we will approach them as if they are until they prove otherwise.

Values

These are the moral principles, beliefs or accepted standards of individuals or groups. For example, we may value honesty, friendships or family life.

Our beliefs, values and attitudes influence how we behave towards others and can also lead us to form prejudices.

Prejudice and discrimination

Prejudice

These are pre-formed views about something, someone or a group of people. They are usually unfavourable, such as a dislike or intolerance for people with certain characteristics, and are usually based not on facts but on incomplete information or stereotypes which highlight people's assumed characteristics. They can be influenced by other people's views or the information we receive through family, friends or the media.

Discrimination

This results when we put our prejudices into action in a way which treats some individuals less favourably than others.

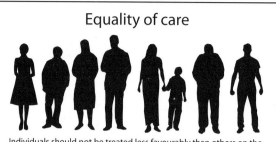

Fig. 3.2   Equality of care.

Prejudice or discrimination can be directed against anyone but most often targets minority groups within a society. Common prejudices are racism, ageism, sexism and homophobia. Other categories which can form the basis of discrimination are shown in Fig. 3.2.

Discrimination can occur in a range of ways, for example:

- Age barriers, e.g. people over 70 are not invited for jury service and have to apply for a driving licence every year
- Organisations refusing admission on the grounds of gender, race or religion
- Buildings with no access for wheelchair users
- Health promotion literature in English only, rather than a range of languages appropriate to a multi-cultural society
- Information not offered in large print and Braille for people with visual impairment, and audiotapes for people with hearing impairment
- Images showing only white, young, able-bodied, heterosexual people, rather than from all races, age groups and abilities, and including some same-sex couples

Rights and responsibilities

Rights

Rights are entitlements which should morally, ethically, legally or fairly belong to an individual. Few rights are absolute or timeless. Most exist in a relationship with others and insofar as they are granted by those around us. In Western society fundamental rights are the right to life, freedom of speech, freedom to live without violence and right to clean air and water. Children and young adolescents have additional rights to care and protection.

Rights within health and social care include:

- Receiving health care on the basis of clinical need, regardless of ability to pay
- Being registered with a general practitioner (GP) and referred to a consultant when the GP thinks appropriate

- Receiving emergency medical care at any time
- Receiving a clear explanation of any treatment proposed, including any risks and alternatives
- Having access to health records and for these to be treated confidentially

Users of care services have rights including the right to be:

- Recognised and cared for as an individual in a humane way
- Respected for one's culture and religious beliefs
- Respected for one's lifestyle and relationships
- Given respect for privacy and dignity
- Able to make choices and have those choices respected
- Safe and secure
- Free to move around and spend one's time as one chooses
- Helped to remain as healthy and independent as possible

An important right in everyday caring situations is that clients give informed consent to the treatment and care they are offered. In other words, are they happy for you to do what you are doing in the way in which you are doing it? Have they received full explanations and given all the options? Does the individual truly understand all the implications of what is being offered? Being sure that an individual has given informed consent is not always straightforward when the person is very vulnerable, has mental health needs or difficulty in communicating. Consent can be implied, for example if a client holds out his hand to receive a tablet, but this should not be taken for granted. Some people, especially when vulnerable, will be happy to give over control, but great care should be taken to ensure that their right to withdraw consent is upheld. When individuals are unable to advocate for their own rights, relatives or others may advocate for them. Staff sometimes act as advocates for the rights of vulnerable people and advocacy services are available through agencies such as Age Concern.

Another fundamental right in care is confidentiality. This rests on trust and can easily be breached. Clients have the right to believe that the personal information they entrust to care services will only be used for the purpose for which is was intended and will not be given to others without permission. Confidentiality in documentary data must also be protected. If in doubt, seek advice.

Consent and confidentiality are discussed in more detail in Chapter 2.

A range of codes of practice exist to protect people's rights, for example the Code of Professional Practice published by the Nursing and Midwifery Council[3] and the Royal College of Nursing's booklet on guidance on professional matters for carers[4].

Responsibilities

Under law each person has responsibility for him- or herself, unless he or she is mentally ill in a manner which brings them within the scope of mental health legislation. Every member of the caring team has responsibility and accountability to patients, clients and others with whom we work, to ourselves, to our employers and to the organisations within which we work.

Risk

Risk is the possibility of incurring misfortune, loss, damage or danger. Risk can alternatively be viewed as an element of life which adds excitement and, without which, life would be less interesting.

Practice to care

In care settings people can be disadvantaged, discriminated against or have their rights violated in subtle ways, such as:

- Documentation asking for details of husband or wife (thus not acknowledging people who are not married or whose partner is of the same gender)
- No mirrors, sanitary products or condom machines in lavatories for people with disabilities (suggesting the view that such people do not need to see themselves, are not sexual beings and do not wish to have sexual intercourse)
- Pork as the only option on a menu (thus leaving no choice for vegetarians, vegans or people of the Muslim or Jewish faiths who do not eat pork)
- Help with personal care offered only by male care assistants on a shift. This may be unacceptable to women who have never had a male partner or whose religious traditions stipulate that they may be seen naked only by their husbands.

In all care settings clients and staff have both rights and responsibilities, and decisions have to be taken on how these are to be balanced. Working in a hospital, home care service or care home setting brings care workers into contact with relatives as well as clients. In practice, care workers must ensure they remember that clients, if over 18 years of age, can make decisions from themselves and that their relatives may sometimes have different views. Their view may be appropriate, but the care worker has a responsibility to go back to the supervisor and discuss the situation. The supervisor in turn will address the issues and find the best way forward. Clients and relatives have a responsibility to understand that the care worker may not be in a position to change a care arrangement.

Clients have the right to continue to live their lives as they want, and a care worker does not have the right to stop that, unless there has been a legal undertaking to do so, for example a person detained under the Mental Health Act 1983[5], or when an agreement has been reached with the individual and/or the family that staff will manage a particular problem in a certain way. A person who is obese but eats chocolate all day may be advised that this is not a wise activity, but the care worker has no right to remove the chocolate. Equally care workers have the right to refuse to undertake a care activity if they feel, and can demonstrate, that it could damage they health or be dangerous in some way.

Risks need to be assessed throughout the working day in any care setting. Care workers should understand that they have a responsibility to assess for risks when they carry out their work. For example moving a client should not be carried out without a risk assessment. This is done in a few moments by looking at the possible dangers, identifying how to reduce the risks and then using the correct manual handling procedures to carry out the care. Moving and handling are discussed in more detail in Chapter 8.

Care risks will be assessed by the health or social care professionals who are responsible for the person's care, for example risk of falling, pressure damage, using the bath unaided, or leaving a building unescorted. The care worker has a role to play in giving information to the staff about their observations and carrying out the care prescribed. Someone who is at high risk of falling and sustaining a serious injury may need to be supervised constantly while using the toilet. If given this instruction the care worker must carry it out. The risk to the person being left alone is high and the moment the care worker leaves the patient could fall, break a hip and die as a result. Here the care worker has a responsibility to carry out care that has been prescribed. If they disagree, they must discuss their views with senior staff and, until instructed otherwise, continue to deliver the prescribed care.

Summary

In caring for diverse individuals we should celebrate difference, value communities and work with each person in ways which empower and uphold rights.

Diversity encompasses all the ways in which we differ from each other but also, as Beverley Malone suggests[6]:

> the word implies inclusiveness and humanity. It is about the entire community in all its rich variety. Diversity is about respecting difference, rather than seeing difference as a problem or a barrier. Diversity needs to be seen as a series of opportunities and challenges and, above all, as a strength. Our patients, clients and the community we serve benefit when we make diversity mainstream. The more sensitive we are to their differences, the better we get at providing the individualised care that they want and need.

Communities are also important and, particularly when needing care, individuals can gain truly understanding support from those who share their traditions, languages and modes of behaviour. For example, through the Alzheimer's Society telephone helpline for people who are lesbian or homosexual, carers can gain deeply empathic help from a homosexual or lesbian who has experience of a supporting relationship with someone with dementia. Communities can be created and supported by welcoming community members into care services and also through contact with relevant literature or entertainment. Examples include Braille or taped newspapers for people with visual impairment, television programmes such as *See Hear* for the deaf community and publications such as *The Pink Paper* for contact with homosexual or lesbian communities.

Ultimately we should work with individuals in ways which empower them. Language is a powerful tool and, rather than referring to 'the disabled', 'the elderly' or 'the demented' we should value people's uniqueness by referring to them as a person with a disability, an older person or a person living with dementia. Equally we must be vigilant not to disempower people by, for example, 'talking down' to them, restricting their choice or movement for our own convenience, leaving them in nightwear or stained clothes longer than necessary, or infantilising adults with the enforcement of cuddly toys, bibs or nappies.

Those in caring services are privileged to work with an enormously diverse range of individuals who are different from themselves. We have the opportunity to learn so much from their lives, beliefs, traditions and experiences. As Verena Tschudin said: '. . . listening with the whole person . . . is right at the heart of a helping relationship. By listening, we give ourselves to that person at this moment, which is no more and no less than required if we want to help anyone'[7].

References

1. Wedderburn Tate, C. (2003) Beyond the visible. *Diversity in Nursing* **1** (1), 3.
2. White, I. and Heath, H. (2002) Introduction. In: Heath, H., White, I. (eds) *The Challenge of Sexuality in Health Care*. Blackwell, Oxford.
3. Nursing and Midwifery Council (2002) *Code of Professional Conduct*. Nursing and Midwifery Council, London.
4. Royal College of Nursing (2004) *RCN Guidelines on Professional Matters for Health Care Assistants and Nurse Cadets*. Royal College of Nursing, London.
5. Department of Health and Social Security (1983) *Mental Health Act 1983*. HMSO, London.
6. Malone, B. (2003) Inclusiveness and humanity. *Diversity in Nursing* **1** (1), 10.
7. Tschudin, V. (1982) *Counselling Skills for Nurses*. Ballière Tindall, London.

Chapter 4
Communication

Jenny Partridge and Angela Dustagheer

Overview

Communication skills are not only essential but crucial within a carer's role, and interpersonal interaction is of great importance in the caring situation. In this chapter the different methods of communication are discussed with emphasis on verbal and non-verbal methods. The barriers to communication are described, including perception and the environment.

Key words: Verbal; non-verbal; sensory deficit; interpersonal skills; personal presentation; aids to communication; team working; perception; environment

What is communication?

We all talk about communication, but what do we actually mean? To start with, try to define what you mean by communication.

Activity 4.1

Identify six words, which would answer the question: What does communication mean to you?

You may have used words such as:

- Information
- Speaking
- One person to another
- Writing

Let's look at the *Oxford Concise English Dictionary*: 'The action of communicating. The means of sending or receiving information.' This is a broad definition of communication, which is constantly necessary for us to manage our everyday lives. Information can be misunderstood and misinterpreted very easily and the consequences of this can be devastating, especially in the health care environment. Many of the issues arising and complaints made can be traced back to the lack of effective communication and/or interpersonal interaction skills.

When do we start communicating?

Some scientists would say that a baby in the womb is capable of receiving communications and that behaviour patterns after birth reflect messages sent by their mothers. Non-verbal communication is predominant in an infant and the verbal response develops during the second year.

How do we communicate?

Often communication is broken down into two broad categories: verbal and non-verbal.

Activity 4.2

Find some examples of verbal communication.

Communicating: For verbal communication you might have written speech, on the telephone, talking and then got stuck. You might have extended the list to include television and radio. If you thought of verbal as meaning words then your list might suddenly have grown to include newspapers, magazines, letters, telephones, faxes, electronic mail, etc.

The way you speak can be examined in terms of tone, pitch and speed, for example, which are all parts of speech and are called paralinguistics. Also 'hm hm' and 'uh uh' act as reinforcement for communications. All the time words are being delivered as a means of communicating. This may be a two-way communication, such as talking to someone face to face or on the telephone (Fig. 4.1) or one-way, such as looking at the television or reading the newspaper.

Activity 4.3

List some examples of non-verbal communication.

Examples of non-verbal communication you may have identified could be:

- Eye contact
- The distance you stand away from the person with whom you are communicating and whether you are sitting or standing and level with each other

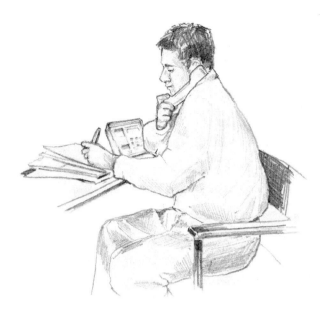

Fig. 4.1   Two-way communication on the telephone. (Adapted from Argyll and Trower, 1979[1]).

- Facial expressions
- Body language, for example, the way you stand, place your hands or arms, gestures
- Touch

In fact these are as important if not more important than the verbal examples, as communication messages are being relayed. As a carer, it is important to be aware that verbal and non-verbal messages must be in agreement. The carer is in a powerful position in relation to the client who may be dependent upon the person giving care. Awareness to equalise the power relationship is necessary, to demonstrate respect of person, maintain dignity and to foster client participation in the care.

Body language

This is a large subject and can be broken down into a number of small areas. The overall picture presented to someone else is very important. The first and last impressions that people have of you are the ones they remember – the primary and recency effects, as psychologists like to call them. Consequently, personal presentation is an important part of communication.

Verbal and non-verbal communications should reflect or reinforce each other. Imagine how you would feel as a client if a carer asked you how you were feeling and they were standing with their arms crossed and did not meet your eye? Or you asked a client how they were feeling and they said fine, but when you observed them they were curled up in bed with downcast eyes showing that the verbal and non-verbal messages were not in agreement. In both these examples two different messages are being given.

What sort of impression do you wish to give to your client? The position of our bodies is most important and will communicate a great deal to our companion(s). If someone is leaning forward it tends to signify interest or encouragement, whilst leaning backwards could be interpreted as boredom or disinterest, or, on the other hand, extreme relaxation. Equally, crossed arms may indicate a lack of interest and not wishing to get involved, even though it may be a cold day and you are trying to keep warm! These closed signals can also indicate a wish to terminate the conversation as quickly as possible and go on to something else.

Eye contact

Lovers are described as 'gazing into each other's eyes', but too much eye contact can be disconcerting and lead to discomfort on the part of the recipient. The eyes are said to be the 'mirror of the soul' and send messages unconsciously to the other person. When we are listening to someone we tend to maintain eye contact but when we are speaking we tend to have intermittent eye contact and signals can be sent to indicate 'I'm ready to speak or listen' (Fig. 4.2).

Activity 4.4

Without telling a colleague what you are going to do, carry on a conversation with them for two minutes keeping close eye contact. Then continue the conversation with them for another two minutes deliberately avoiding any eye contact. How do you both feel at the end?

Probably your colleague will ask what on earth you were doing, but will also say that they felt quite threatened in the first exercise and it was difficult to keep

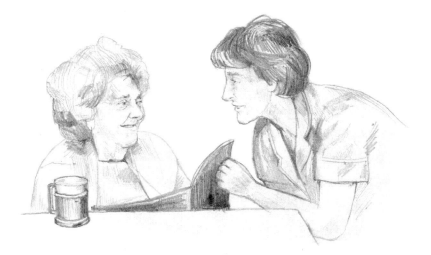

Fig. 4.2   Maintaining eye contact. (Adapted from Argyll and Trower, 1979[1]).

the conversation going. In the second the comments may well be that you appeared disinterested and weren't really concerned with what was being said.

Eye contact can reinforce the messages we send. However, it may have particular significance in different cultures. In some cultures it is considered discourteous to look someone in the eye if they are older or wiser than yourself.

Position and space

Linked to eye contact is the comparative position we place ourselves in to communicate.

Activity 4.5

Try placing yourself in different positions relative to your colleague and carry on a conversation. These positions may be, for example side by side, one standing and one sitting, back to back, very close together or wide apart. You will probably think of more. Which was the easiest position to converse?

You will probably have found sitting nearly opposite each other the easiest and the distance may well reflect the length of time you have known each other. The better we know a person the nearer we let them come to us. We have an 'intimate area' which is approximately 45 cm around us (Fig. 4.3), a 'personal area' from there to about 1.2 m, then a 'social area' of 3.7 m and finally a public area from there onwards[2].

On the whole we do not allow anyone to violate our personal space (see Activity 4.5) or we have strict conditions if this happens. As carers we have to gain permission to enter that intimate zone as so much of our care is very personal and does in fact violate that space.

Activity 4.6

When you are in a queue, for example waiting for a bus or at a check-out in a supermarket, see what happens if you edge forward nearer the person in front. Be careful about the supermarket trolleys!

The chances are that the person you tried to get nearer to tried to move away and keep the ratio of space the same. You may also have been the recipient of some fairly foul glances as well – another method of non-verbal communication and protection of space.

Relative position

This is also important in the physical levels of people; if one person is much higher than the other it can be seen as a commanding position and the lower

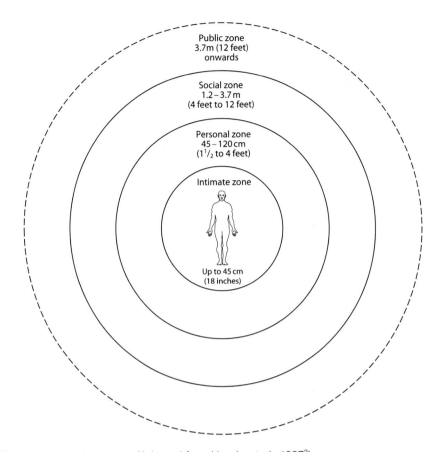

Fig. 4.3 Interaction zones. (Adapted from Hargie *et al.*, 1987[2]).

person feels at a disadvantage. It can also hinder or facilitate any contact and effective communication.

We can also send messages to the client by changing our relative position. For example, if we sit down to talk to a client we are telling them we have time and will concentrate on them for that specific time. Communication can be:

$A \rightarrow B$ one-way or
$A \leftarrow B / A \rightarrow B$ two-way.

In the carer–client relationship it is important to ensure that communication remains two-way and the client is listened to effectively. It is easy in this relationship for the carer to assume a powerful position and the communication may become one-way. Clients should feel able to express themselves and articulate their needs. Within the duty of care framework, the carer should listen closely to what the client says and include them in the process of care planning.

Language

Language is used in different ways, as is choice of words; it is context specific.

Activity 4.7

Think of the different types of television programmes that you watch – news, sports programmes, soap operas, documentaries, gardening or home improvement programmes. How does the language differ in these programmes?

Your observation might include that the language in the news bulletin is formal and more complex words may be used. Each soap opera is different – the characters may speak in dialect and use different words. In programmes for young children, there may be an emphasis on non-verbal communication backed up with visual aids, usually with the use of bright colours.

Tone of voice, intonation and how words are emphasised can convey messages; they can hinder or improve communication. Many of the issues and complaints that arise in care stem from a lack of effective communicative and interpersonal interaction skills. In everyday adult conversations, there is not always a commitment to actively listen to what the other person is actually saying. Assumptions are made and there is often a tendency to interrupt to make a point. In care, it is important to become self-aware of one's communication style and to develop skills to actively listen and be empathetic to the other person.

Gestures

These are often used to emphasise points. Some people use gestures more than others, and continue to gesture to emphasise points when they are on the telephone, even though their listener cannot see them. On the other hand gestures can also signal what the body really feels rather than what is being said[1]. If you watch someone who is being interviewed they may appear calm and say they are not worried, but in fact they are fiddling with something or crossing and uncrossing their legs all the time. So messages may be contrary in their presentation and the true reaction has to be found for effective communication to take place (Fig. 4.4).

Smiling and nodding one's head are gestures of encouragement to others to continue to talk. Smiling alters the tone of the voice and it is suggested that you should smile whilst answering the telephone as it sounds better at the other end. It will give confidence to someone to continue and put over their point of view. It also reinforces the fact that you are interested and listening to the client. A useful way you can remember this is 'SOLER'[3]:

Smile, sit facing the other person
Open manner, arms by one's side

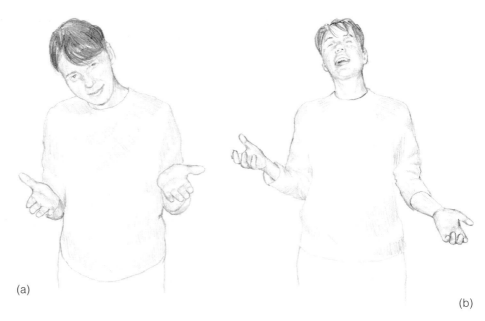

(a)

(b)

Fig. 4.4   Gestures of communication. (a) Offer. (b) Laugh.

Lean slightly forward – NB: remember leaning too far forward may be inter-
    preted as an aggressive move
Eye contact
Relax, respond

Touch

There are times when it may be said that gestures speak louder than words. The
way we handle or touch clients can be a positive way of communication and our
attitude can be portrayed in the way we may lift a client's leg when washing or
turning them. I am sure when you have felt upset someone may have just
touched your arm or squeezed your hand as no words are necessary to tell you
that the other person cares. This applies to the majority of people but it is important to be aware that some people do not like to be touched and like to retain a
distance of several metres. From the carer's point of view it is important you feel
comfortable with this aspect of care, otherwise you may look awkward and it
will have the opposite effect.

Barriers to communication

Having reviewed different methods of communication we can see where problems may arise in messages and intentions being understood and acted upon
appropriately. The saying goes that, 'You can take a horse to the water but you
cannot make it drink'.

The same is true for communication; you can tell someone something but they may not act upon it for a variety of reasons; it may be a simple reason of not hearing and a straight repetition will ensure the intended response. Or the reasons may be more complex. An individual may also only hear what they wish to hear – this is known as selective listening. The hearer may filter out what is painful or stressful to know and they may not want to act on that communication, so even if they hear the words they won't do anything about it deliberately. Anxiety may also interfere with the amount of information received and understood.

There may be a physical reason for a communication gap. Sensory deprivation such as blindness, deafness, learning difficulties or illness may lead to communication barriers. The UK is a multi-cultural society and there may be a language barrier if English is the second language or the person may not speak any English at all.

Blindness

Activity 4.8

If you have the opportunity at work, with a partner, take turns in putting a blindfold on and being moved around by the 'sighted' partner.

You probably felt very disorientated despite the fact you thought you knew where you were, and you asked a great many questions of your partner about where you were and where pieces of furniture were. In communication we use a number of senses to understand messages and once we lose one of those senses we need additional information and reassurance to maintain the same level of understanding. You may have heard someone say 'I need my glasses, I cannot understand what you are saying.'

Deafness

Activity 4.9

Again, working with a partner, ensure they cannot hear by using a personal stereo or equivalent and then ask them to undertake a simple task such as moving a book from one table to another, by gesture and demonstrating. How successful is the 'deaf' person?

Hearing loss is often described as the invisible disability as people look normal but appear to have difficulty in comprehending information. It therefore becomes an enormous communication barrier unless people adapt their behaviour to cope with this, and the affected individual may get frustrated and lose self-esteem. People with hearing loss have to concentrate very hard to pick up all the cues and sounds to make sense of what is being said to them. This can lead to tiredness and frustration. A carer should give information in stages and allow for natural breaks. Giving too much information at once can overwhelm the person with hearing loss, and it is useful to back up information with written details so that the client can read this later on. This helps to reduce the client's anxiety and promotes communication. When the client has had a chance to read the written details, then time should be allowed for any questions to be asked.

If people suffer hearing loss, in addition to having a hearing aid, learning sign language or how to lip read may help them develop coping strategies for enhancing their level of understanding. If the speaker's face is clearly lit, and turned upwards, this helps the deaf individual to lip read and follow facial expressions. The speaker should also speak clearly and reasonably slowly so that the deaf person has a better chance of hearing. Deaf people often tip their heads in the direction of the speaker to try to hear more clearly and to block out extraneous noise.

Speech disorders

Inability to speak is another barrier to communication. This could, for example, be due to a stroke resulting in dysphasia (difficulty in speaking), or cerebral palsy. There are many clients who have a speech disorder and who may exhibit great frustration in attempting to communicate. The speech therapist plays an important role in assessing and treating these clients, exercises may be given and the carer may be involved in this process.

Learning difficulties and language barriers

Barriers are evident if people have learning difficulties. As we develop, our brain's ability to understand and comprehend expands. It is beyond a child's capability to understand what time is until they have learned to tell the time. Even so, communication has to be altered for them to understand, so as adults we are guilty of saying to clients that we will be there 'in a minute' whilst there is not the slightest chance that we can be there in a quarter of an hour.

As a carer it is important to make an effort to communicate directly with any client who has communication problems. Time should be spent to find out what is being said and it may be necessary to use communication aids. With clients who have communication problems, speech should be clear and direct. The carer should use plain English, and jargon, technical terms and abbreviations should be avoided or, if used, an explanation should be given. The person being cared for would ideally be given a chance to absorb information, preferably backed up with written materials and then given the opportunity later to ask questions. It may be appropriate to go over the information a second time.

Communication then has to reflect the common ground and abilities between the parties involved and sometimes this requires the asking of questions to identify the common ground. The use of language varies from limited to extended. At times limited language may be necessary, for example, if someone is in danger we may just call out 'Stop', but if there is no danger and we want someone's attention to talk to them we may say, 'Hang on a minute will you, I'd like to have a word.'

Questioning

Activity 4.10

Write down all the types of, or ways of, asking questions you can think of.

Your list may be probably quite extensive and include the following:

- Open
- Factual
- Clarifying
- Leading
- Closed
- Rhetorical
- Multiple

There is a place for all these types of question in communication, but they must be used in the appropriate way to be effective and careful thought must be given before using the last two (multiple or rhetorical), as they either confuse or control communications. By receiving answers to questions it is possible to judge whether communication barriers exist which need to be overcome.

Open questions

This type of question is the preferred mode of questioning as it encourages a full answer. The respondent has a chance to put forward their comments, feelings and opinions and it reflects two-way communication.

Closed questions

These, on the other hand, are used when a brief response is required and may link with factual questions where the questioner is trying to elicit responses for factual purposes. These are usually answered by a 'Yes' or a 'No'.

Rhetorical questions

These are used when it could be thought that the client wants to talk more, and by repeating the statement in a questioning manner it may trigger the respondent to speak further.

Clarifying questions

These may use the same structure to ensure that the person asking the question and the respondent are talking about the same thing and putting similar meanings to the subject. It is important at times to check out with the client that you have understood. For example, the carer can respond, 'I understand that you are saying' and repeat what the client has said.

Multiple questions

These are very tempting to ask, especially if there is a time constraint involved. However, it is very difficult for the respondent to reply as there is a large degree of uncertainty as to which answer belongs to which question; and for most of us our short-term memory will not hold all the information. The situation is also made worse if the client is anxious, ill or confused.

Leading questions

These tend to invite a specific answer and the respondent may feel under pressure to give the expected answer rather than the one they really want to give. These questions can be used when enquiring about someone's well-being. For instance we may say 'Feeling all right are you?' and the expected answer is 'Yes, thank you'. In care it is often crucial to obtain information from the client's point of view and therefore this type of questioning has limited or no use in care settings.

Language

The variety of languages encountered in our society today means that we require either an excellent interpreting service or some other means of making sure we are communicating effectively. Language cards are one solution, and language cards with pictures are even better, given the wide variety of dialects involved.

Even in the English language the meaning of a word can differ in different parts of the country and different words can be used to describe even the most simple of actions. It is a challenge to find the appropriate word, but much distress can be avoided if these differences are recognised early. Not only is language different, but gestures which are quite usual and normal in one country may be perceived as rude and insulting in another. For example, in the Middle East, it is considered polite to burp at the end of a meal to signify appreciation of the food you have eaten; not to burp is an insult to the host.

Colloquial expressions also cause difficulties for people learning English as a second language. How many times have you asked someone to 'hang on' at the other end of the telephone? Hang on to what?

Every type of work has its own jargon; perhaps in the caring services we have more than most, or perhaps our time is at a premium so we use jargon as a short cut. Whatever the reason, it does mean that everyone should have an understanding of what the jargon actually means, but preferably for reasons of safety, it should be used as little as possible.

Activity 4.11

Make a list of all the jargon terms you can find in your place of work.

No examples are going to be given here, but do you truly know the meaning of all the words in *your* list? If not, ask at least one other person for their interpretation or definitions. You may be very surprised how different they are from your understanding. In the interests of clarity and safety try to avoid the use of jargon and use plain English.

As an individual every client will have different communication needs. As a carer you will need to use your skills to find the most appropriate and effective methods of communicating with your clients. Equally, you have a responsibility to communicate with your colleagues in the care team. Team work is composed of a great many lines of communication and if these are broken or inadequately maintained misinterpretation occurs and wrong messages may get through.

Activity 4.12

Make a list of all the team members with whom you communicate during a span of duty.

You may only have a small list if you work mainly on your own or in a small group. However, if you work in a large busy hospital you may have a very long list. With your list, can you recollect an incident where the communication was effective and an incident where the communication was ineffective? Compare the differences. In your answer, was the communication effectiveness linked to clarity of speech or use of jargon? Was it clearly understood or misinterpreted? Was there good listening or not listening or denial of facts, or matching understanding of a word or different understanding of a word meaning? It is crucial that we check with the client that our understanding of words and language match.

Other factors affecting communication

Physical/psychological

How we are feeling at any one time will affect communication. If you are happy then you feel like chatting freely; however, if you are in pain or discomfort then you may not feel like talking to anyone at all.

Perception

This is our personal understanding or interpretation and it is dependent on previous experiences. Perception is two-way and while we perceive the person with whom we are communicating, they perceive us. There are times when we need to check our perception. For instance, if we see someone curled up in bed looking unhappy, we may wish to check by asking 'How are you feeling?', or by saying 'I get the impression that you're feeling fed up and may be in some sort of discomfort'. Hopefully this will let the client know that you are receiving their message and are concerned about them and it will usually precipitate a response, which can lead to your knowing more about them, how they feel and their anxieties and concerns.

Environment

The overall environment can either inhibit or facilitate communication.

Activity 4.13

List factors in the environment that could inhibit communication.

Your list may include the following:

- Noise
- Table in between two people
- Seating arrangement
- Lack of privacy

This could be quite an extensive list as many factors interfere with effective communication.

Activity 4.14

List factors in the environment that could facilitate communication.

The factors could include:

- Comfortable chairs set an angle and at the same height
- Phone switched to answerphone mode
- Giving the client full attention
- Soft light
- Quietness

Summary

This chapter has looked at communication. Consider the activities you have completed. You are now ready to look for opportunities to enhance your communication skills in all aspects of caring.

References

1. Argyle, M. and Tower, P. (1979) *Person to Person; Ways of Communicating.* Harper & Row, London.
2. Hargie, O., Saunders, C. and Dickson, D. (1987) *Social Skills in Interpersonal Communication.* Croom Helm, London.
3. Egan, G. (1985) *The Skilled Helper, A Systematic Approach to Effective Helping.* Brooks/ Cole Publishing Company, California.

Further reading

Brewin, T. and Sporshott, M. (1996) *Relating to Relatives. Breaking Bad News Communication and Support.* Radcliffe Medical Press, Oxford.

Burnard, P. (1994) *Effective Communication Skills for Health Professionals.* Chapman Hall, London.

Carr, S. (2002) *Tackling NHS Jargon: Getting the Message Across.* Radcliffe Medical Press, Oxford.

Darley, M. (ed.) (2002) *Managing Communication in Health Care.* Bailliere Tindall in association with the Royal College of Nursing, London.

Faulkner, A. (1997) *Effective Interaction with Patients,* 2nd edition. Churchill Livingstone, Edinburgh.

Middleton, J. (2000) *Primary Care: The Team Guide to Communication.* Radcliffe Medical Press, Oxford.

Niven, N. (2000) *Health Psychology for Health Care Professionals,* 3rd edition. Churchill Livingstone, Edinburgh, pp. 7–28.

Russell, G. (1999) *Essential Psychology for Nurses and other Health Professionals.* Routledge, London.

Chapter 5
Working with people whose behaviour challenges the service

Caroline Coleman

Overview

This chapter will consider behaviour that challenges us in the workplace. It will explore some of the options available to the individual when faced with this behaviour, as well as some guidance about how and why difficult or challenging behaviour occurs. The chapter identifies the importance of recording and reporting incidents and provides the reader with options for further reading to support underpinning knowledge.

Key words: Behaviour; feelings; reactions; cause; trigger; recording; policies; procedures; observation; debrief; awareness; limitations

What is difficult or challenging behaviour?

We are all individuals and so our perception of behaviour that is either difficult or challenging will differ from person to person. Our responses and coping mechanisms may also differ depending on our mood, the environment and how well we know the individual who is challenging us. What may appear to be trivial to one person may well be extremely uncomfortable to another. The experience, knowledge and training of each team member will define the outcome of their response to each challenging incident. For this reason the terms 'difficult' and 'challenging' may be any behaviour that makes us feel uncomfortable, worried or frightened.

Activity 5.1

Describe one example of a recent incident in which you experienced behaviour which you felt was difficult or challenging.

Here are some examples of difficult or challenging behaviour:

- When out shopping, the shop assistant ignored me.
- On my way home from work, I bumped into a man walking along the road and he swore at me.
- Yesterday morning, when I was serving breakfast, a service user threw her cereal at me.

Each team member will have different experiences, knowledge and training in caring for individuals presenting with challenging behaviour. It is important to remember this fact as you develop confidence and knowledge in dealing with difficult situations. Supporting other team members who have found an incident difficult is a key role. Your organisation will have formal methods of supporting care staff who have found incidents difficult. However, individuals providing *ad hoc* support to their colleagues are just as important components in managing the aftermath of an incident as that of the formal process. It is important, therefore, that neither is overlooked.

Within the care sector, the level of challenging and difficult behaviour can be, to some degree, predicted. Care staff who work in units where service users are known to be challenging will receive more intensive training. They may be provided with personal alarms or other safety equipment. The building may have been specifically designed and have reinforced windows or unbreakable mirrors. Within these units, each individual service user's care plan will reflect this level of challenge and care staff will be able to read management guidelines and risk assessments. The role of the carers is therefore to familiarise themselves with the individual service user's care plan.

Where challenging or difficult behaviour is less predictable, care staff may find themselves in a position of risk. As the behaviour may not have been predictable, the response from care staff may be inappropriate. Adequate preparation and training is essential to ensure that care staff become competent at assessing a situation and consequently act appropriately when a problem occurs. Each member of staff has a responsibility to attend training where offered and to read local policies available. Each of us has a responsibility to ensure that we are up to date with our organisation's expectations of dealing with difficult and challenging behaviour. Care staff who fail to do this may place themselves, their colleagues or the service user at further risk[1].

Why does behaviour become difficult or challenging?

There are many factors that may *trigger* challenging behaviour and usually in the course of our work we will not witness the *cause* of the behaviour. The cause is the underlying reason why an individual is likely to present with challenging behaviour. The trigger is the factor that initiates the actual behaviour.

The causes and triggers are often confused, but it is important that we understand the differences, as our own behaviour could be a trigger to a challenging incident.

Activity 5.2

To help differentiate between cause and trigger here is an example. To test your understanding, write down the causes and triggers that may have been present in this scenario.

Joanne's mother is on a hospital waiting list for a hip replacement operation. Her mother's quality of life is significantly reduced and Joanne is very worried about her. This morning she has spoken with the consultant's secretary to see where her mother is on the waiting list. She is told that the secretary is unavailable and that she cannot speak to another appointments clerk, as they are all very busy. Later in the day Joanne goes to the same hospital to find out the results of some recent blood tests. She waits in the queue for some time and eventually is at the front of the queue. A nurse comes over to the booking clerk and discusses the film she saw last night. Although the conversation is brief and lasts only ten seconds, Joanne shouts at the clerk, demanding immediate attention and when the nurse leans forward towards Joanne and says, 'There is no need to be rude,' Joanne swears at the nurse and storms off.

It is important to note that, although the actions of the nurse and the clerk may have represented the trigger for Joanne's outburst, it is unlikely that the clerk or the nurse could have known the cause.

The causes and triggers of challenging behaviour fall into three main categories: physical, psychological and environmental. Examples are given in Table 5.1 under each heading.

How can we predict and avoid difficult or challenging behaviour?

The answer is that we can't predict all behaviour that could be challenging or difficult, nor can we avoid all such behaviour. What we can do is be realistic about the likelihood of challenging or difficult behaviour occurring. We can also be aware of the likely causes and triggers of such behaviour and we can recognise individuals who are presenting us with indications that they are not comfortable.

All services are now risk assessed[2]. Risk is the likelihood that actual harm will occur. A hazard is something with the potential to do harm. This means that each workplace has both generic and specific risk assessments. These are documents which calculate the likelihood of risk, categorise the risk and score the risk. Risk

Table 5.1 Causes/triggers of difficult behaviour.

Physical	Psychological	Environmental
Pain	Emotional upsets	Room temperature
Dietary factors	Stress	Unjustified restrictions
Alcohol/drugs	Tension	Noise
Hunger/thirst	Confusion	Unknown surroundings
Hormonal	Frustration	Unfamiliar people
Clinical conditions	Powerlessness	Others' behaviour
Shock	Mental health	Routine changes
No verbal communication	History of abuse	Smoky atmosphere

assessments are used in all parts of our work, as required under the Management of Health and Safety at Work Regulations 1992[3]. This legislation places a general requirement on employers to assess all risks involved in their work activity. Where there is a significant risk, this assessment must be recorded.

Generic risk assessments should be completed for hazards or activities that are common throughout the department. Specific assessments should be completed for particular tasks, procedures, equipment, locations, etc. which have specific significant risks.

The essential steps taken by individual work places in order to comply with these regulations are to:

- Identify the hazards to health or safety arising from the activity or the workplace
- Decide who might be harmed and how
- Evaluate the risks and decide whether existing precautions are adequate or more needs to be done
- Record your findings
- Review your assessment and revise if necessary

An example of a completed risk assessment form is given in Fig. 5.1. It is usual for a senior or experienced member of staff to complete the risk assessment. However, the assessor may request information from you personally, as you may have more knowledge of the workplace activity than they have. Some workplaces have trained assessors to carry out this task. Your employer is responsible for carrying out a risk assessment and they will review the risk on a regular, pre-determined basis.

Activity 5.3

Consider one of your normal duties at work and write down a list of existing control measures which are in place to reduce risk. You may be surprised at how much risk has already been reduced in your workplace.

One of the control measures used in protecting the receptionist (see Fig. 5.1) was her knowledge and recent training. It is possible that she received training in recognising the signs or signals that individuals may present. The most obvious signs that an individual is upset, happy, angry or confused are those of body language and facial expression. These are usually linked to verbal communication, where the individual verbally expresses his or her happiness, anger or confusion (see Chapter 4). However, this is not always the case and individuals who are feeling threatened, confused or anxious may not verbally convey what they are feeling (Fig. 5.2).

Activity 5.4

Make a list of signs which may indicate that a client's level of anger is increasing.

Risk assessment

Department: GP surgery   **Actions required**   Yes/~~No~~

Assessor: Jean Nicholson   **Date:** 3 April 2002

Job title: Receptionist   **Location:** Office Area

Hazard: Assault from patients   **Line manager:** Dr. S. R. Macklam

---

Known accident/incidents

In March 2001
December 2001
Both occasions, patients became angry at having to wait for an appointment and grabbed the receptionist by the collar/throat area

---

Existing controls	Control effectiveness
Glass fronted reception area	H
Training and experience of receptionist in dealing with difficult behaviour	H
Posters informing patients of appointment system	M
Feedback/communication system for patients	L
Community liaison with local police officers	M
Telephone beside reception desk	H

Conclusions

Since the changes were made to the surgery and training given to the receptionist, the likelihood of repetition has been reduced. A further review will be needed on a monthly basis, so that further consideration may be given

---

Actions identified

All actions taken as identified in staff meeting, however, further staff training and improved communication systems may be needed and therefore this risk assessment will be reviewed each month at the staff meeting

---

Hazard likelihood	Severity/consequences	Control effectiveness
1. Highly unlikely	1. Negligible injuries	H High
2. Remote possible	2. Minor injuries	M Medium
3. Occasional occurrence	3. Major injuries	L Low
4. Fairly frequent	4. Single fatality	
5. Frequent and regular	5. Multiple fatalities	
6. Almost certainly	6. Multiple fatalities (inc off site)	

Fig. 5.1 An example of a completed risk assessment form.

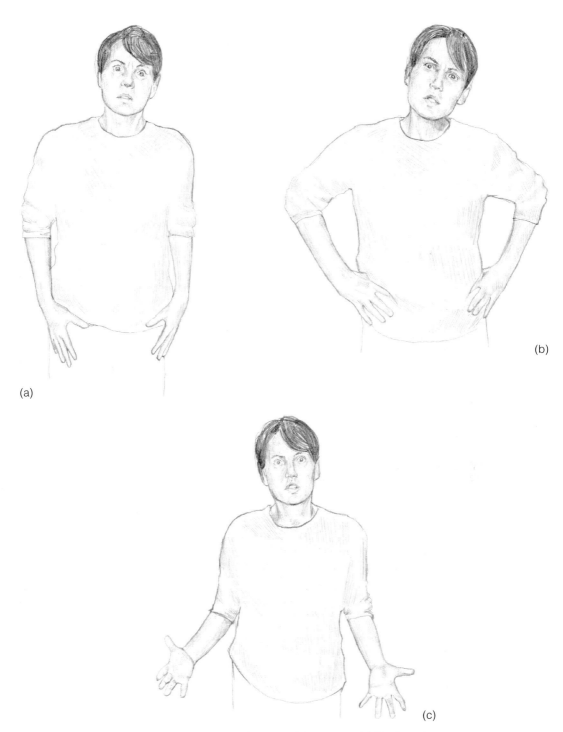

Fig. 5.2   Visual indications of (a) mood (b) anger and (c) indignation.

Your list may include:

- Tension and body posture
- Grim facial expression
- Increased volume and rate of speech
- Clenched fists
- Grinding of teeth
- Abusive language
- Violent behaviour

Observation of potentially difficult service users

If you are caring for a service user who you know has difficult or challenging behaviour and you are not sure what is causing this, in preparation for future incidents, it is likely that you or other colleagues may be asked to observe the service user. It is usual that this is a specific piece of work and is time limited.

There are several ways to observe people. The most obvious way is just to keep a close eye on them, but the results may be influenced by the individual team member's own perception. For example, a service user may regularly request that their visitors leave soon after they arrive. The individual team member may decide that the service user is happier on his or her own, or that as a result of the service user's hearing problem he or she becomes confused by the complexity of conversations. In reality, if the team member stayed in the area long enough to see what happens after the service user's request for the visitors to leave, the team member would see the service user going to watch his or her favourite television programme.

The most reliable way is to use a recognised and agreed observation tool. Staff members must never record observed behaviours without prior agreement. It is accepted practice that the recording of observed behaviour will be carried out under supervision by senior members of the team and with agreement with all disciplines who have responsibility for the individual service user's care.

The observation chart most commonly used and recognised is the ABC chart (Table 5.2) which is based on:

A: Antecedent: what happened before the incident
B: Behaviour: what behaviour was observed
C: Consequence: what happened immediately after the incident

From the observations recorded on the form, team members might see a pattern emerge. It may be that the information collected is seen by a psychologist who will support team members in understanding the information collected.

Table 5.2   ABC observation chart (adapted from *STEP Manual*[4]).

Date/time	Antecedent	Behaviour	Consequence	Signature

The importance of recording the consequence of an incident is that team members can assess whether or not a pattern emerges around this time to support the behaviour. For example, each time a child has a temper tantrum a mother may give the child a sweet. The reason the mother gives the child a sweet is to curtail the undesirable behaviour. However, the longer-term consequences of this action may reinforce the negative behaviour and thus teach the child to repeat the undesirable behaviour.

Dealing with difficult behaviour

The best method of dealing with difficult or challenging behaviour is to make sure that you are well prepared before the incident occurs. Take some time to think about how prepared you would be in dealing with a difficult situation. Listed below are some guidelines to help you prepare.

- Familiarise yourself with your organisation's procedures, including those for when you are working away from your base or with colleagues from other organisations. Find out if there are systems in place to alert colleagues when you are in difficulty.
- Understand what triggers violence and abuse, so that you are prepared to cope with violence and abuse which may occur in your job. Be aware of your approach and the effect it may have on others.
- Read the procedures for raising any concerns you have with colleagues and managers.
- When you think there is a risk, discuss your concerns with colleagues and managers. Whenever possible get to know the service user. Make time to read service users' admission or care plan documents.
- Gather as much information as possible about threatening service users and share it with your colleagues and manager.
- Attend training that promotes safer practice.

What to do when an incident occurs

However well prepared you may be, unpredictable or difficult behaviour may still occur. Faced with difficult situations, you should not let the situation escalate until it becomes unmanageable. There are two ways to respond appropriately:

- manage the incident
- summon help

The option you choose will depend upon a number of factors, such as how competent you feel about dealing with the situation, the amount of support around you, how well you know the service user and how familiar you are with local policies and procedures.

Managing the incident

There are a number of methods which may be effective. Faced with an aggressive person, you should first be aware of yourself. Your body language and voice should be calm and non-threatening and you should not invade the person's personal space. Retain an open, non-aggressive stance. Think about the way you are responding to the person and how you communicate with them. Do not allow the person to think that you are going to take direct aggressive action against them or they will feel threatened.

You must never threaten or challenge the person or defend situations/people that the person is feeling angry about. Do not ridicule or belittle the client, but show respect for him or her even if the individual is not showing it for you. Accept the full verbal expression of angry feelings (swearing will not hurt you) and, whenever possible, remove bystanders or provide an environment where the service user may feel less threatened or more comfortable. Most important of all:

> Don't take chances; don't get hurt; know your limitations

Summon help

Either go to get help or use the systems available to you to summon help. Make sure that you are already aware of the local policies and procedures for getting help. Never feel that you did not do your job properly, for we all have limitations and unfamiliar situations to deal with. If you accept these limitations and seek help, you are dealing with the situation in the most competent and professional way.

Sometimes behaviour becomes so difficult to manage that the service user must be dealt with by other professional bodies. This may include police authorities. Sometimes the behaviour is a result of a mental health problem and therefore a more appropriately trained professional will need to be called upon to assess and/or manage the situation.

After the incident

After the incident has occurred you may experience many forms of emotion. Many people feel upset or worried that they may have caused the problems; others may feel angry or tired. Whatever your feelings are about the situation it is important to recognise that it is a natural response and that the emotions you are experiencing should not be ignored.

Your workplace will have policies and procedures that minimise the harmful impact on the staff member and diminish the risk of repetition. These policies and procedures are often referred to as 'debriefing' or sometimes as critical incident debriefing or post-incident support. This process includes structured time with colleagues and/or senior staff in order to share your experiences or feelings (Fig 5.3). It may be that other facilities are available in your workplace for you to talk about the incident. These may include occupational health,

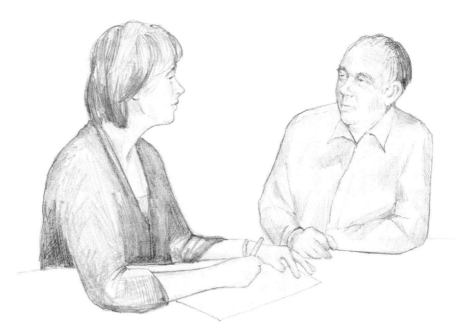

Fig. 5.3 Talking about experiences after an incident.

counselling services or sometimes welfare officers. It may be that there are other support groups in your workplace. Take advantage of these facilities:

- Talk to your colleagues
- Talk to your manager/supervisor
- Share your experiences
- Share feelings

Recording and reporting

As soon as possible after the incident, a full and accurate report should be made to the appropriate person(s) and entered into the records. Your organisation will have specifically designed forms for this purpose. The longer the period between the incident and the writing of the report, the more likely it is that the facts will become confused. Therefore, it should be re-emphasised that report writing occur as soon as possible.

Important facts to record:

- Name of person
- Date and time of incident
- Description of the behaviour observed
- What happed immediately before the incident
- Length of incident
- What happened immediately after the incident
- Any other relevant information

It is important to record the incident, whether a singular event or regular occurrence. These incidents are all of equal importance, as they will affect the care and treatment prescribed for the client and influence preventive actions to be taken against future outbursts.

If an injury has been sustained this must be reported as this is a legal requirement. This requirement is detailed under Reporting of Injuries, Diseases and Dangerous Occurrences Regulations 1995, sometimes referred to as RIDDOR. The information enables the Health and Safety Executive (HSE) and local authorities to identify where and how risks arise and to investigate incidents.

Sometimes the management of a difficult incident will be investigated by your organisation. This may be as a result of a complaint or concern about the seriousness of the incident or perhaps a staff member's practice. Whatever the reason, the clearer the record made, the easier it is for others to establish the facts.

Activity 5.5

Find out what procedure you should follow if you have been injured. Locate and read any forms that would need completion if you have been injured.

Case study

Pam has arrived at your workplace for an appointment with your manager. Your manager has been called away to an urgent meeting and will not be able to see Pam for another hour. Pam appears upset on arrival and sits outside the manager's office. When you attempt to explain the delay, Pam becomes flushed and starts to shake. She attempts to enter the manager's office. The door is locked. When she realises the door is locked she begins to hammer on the door and to shout.

Activity 5.6

How would you attempt to manage this situation? Try to use the option 'Managing the incident', described earlier. You may find it helpful to discuss this exercise with a colleague(s).

There is no correct answer, but by using the guidelines listed earlier under 'What to do if an incident occurs', you should be able to think through some approaches and thus be better equipped to defuse such a situation effectively.

Legal considerations

Each organisation is obliged by law to consider the safety and rights of both the service provider (staff/team member) and the service user (client). Listed below are some of the Acts and conventions that are implemented in your workplace.

- Health and Safety at Work Act 1974
- Crime and Disorder Act 1998
- Sex Discrimination Act 1975
- RIDDOR 1995
- Disability Discrimination Act 1995
- Race Relations Discrimination Act 1976
- Mental Health Act 1983
- Convention for the Protection of Human Rights and Fundamental Freedoms 1950
- Human Rights Act 1998

The Human Rights Act 1998 incorporates the European Convention on Human Rights into UK law. The European Convention on Human Rights was drawn up soon after World War II and the rights and the language used reflect this. There are several Articles which are the standards by which we are required to practice.

Article 8 specifies that:

> Everyone has the right to respect for his private and family life, his home and his correspondence.
>
> There shall be no interference by a public authority with the exercise of this right except in accordance with the law and is necessary in a democratic society in the interest of national security, public safety or the economic well-being of the country, for the prevention of disorder or crime, for the protection of health or morals, or for the protection of the rights and freedoms of others.

Organisations have a responsibility to ensure that the interventions they undertake when dealing with difficult or challenging service users take into account an individual's rights. Observing an individual's behaviour may seem to be an appropriate undertaking and reasonable in assessing risk in the workplace, but this must be balanced and proportionate in the response to a situation or risk.

Summary

Now that you have worked through this chapter and completed all the activities, you should have an increased awareness of yourself, your colleagues and your organisation's responsibilities regarding difficult or challenging behaviour. Remember the key points:

- Don't take chances, don't get hurt
- Become aware of your limitations
- Read the policies and procedures
- Prepare well

- Find out where to get help
- Attend training events you are offered
- Discuss incidents with others
- Record and report appropriately

You may find it helpful to visit some areas to observe experts dealing with difficult behaviour every day. Once you have done this, try looking again at the activities in this chapter. You may find that the answers you now give are quite different from your original ones.

References

1. Department of Health (2001) National Task Force on Violence Against Social Care Staff. *A Safer Place.* HMSO, London.
2. Notes to General Risk Assessment Form. University of Edinburgh, Edinburgh.
3. *Management of Health and Safety at Work Regulations 1999.* HMSO, London.
4. Chamberlain, P. *STEP Manual.* The British Association of Behavioural Psychotherapy.

Further reading

Department of Health (1983) *Mental Health Act 1983.* HMSO, London.

Department for Education and Employment (1995) *Disability Discrimination Act 1995.* HMSO, London.

Department of Health (1998) *Human Rights Act 1998.* HMSO, London.

European Convention for the Protection of Human Rights and Fundamental Freedoms, 1950. European Court for Human Rights.

Home Office (1975) *Sex Discrimination Act 1975.* HMSO, London.

Home Office (1976) *Race Relations Discrimination Act 1976.* HMSO, London.

Home Office (1998) *Crime and Disorder Act 1998.* HMSO, London.

Local organisational policies and procedures.

Murphy, G. (1995) Understanding challenging behaviour. In: Emerson, E. McGill, P. and Mansell, J. (eds) *Severe Learning Disabilities and Challenging Behaviours.* Blackwell Synergy, Oxford.

Royal College of Nursing (2004) *RCN Guidelines on Professional Matters for Health Care Assistants and Nurse Cadets.* Royal College of Nursing, London.

Thompson, A. (2000) Family fortunes. *Community Care* 4 October.

UK Health and Safety Executive 1995. *Reporting of Injuries, Diseases and Dangerous Occurrences Regulations 1995* (RIDDOR). Health and Safety Executive, London.

Wills, T. and La Vigna, G. (1985) *Reinforcement Inventory for Adults.* California Institute for Applied Behavior Analysis, California.

Chapter 6
Obtaining and storing client information

Rita Gale

Overview

One of the most important aspects of your work as a carer will involve you in obtaining, inputting and updating information about clients on computer systems and in manual records. It is vital to the delivery of a high-quality service to clients that medical records are accurate, up to date and readily available, when required.

As a carer, you will have direct contact with clients and therefore be able to obtain from them, or their relatives, the required information, for which you will then have responsibility for recording on the computer system or in manual medical records[1].

This chapter guides you through the ways in which you can obtain the information, record, store and retrieve it, and the methods used to manage the hundreds of thousands of client records which accumulate over long periods of time. It also explains the many ways in which the information is used, in addition to those of direct client care. In order to include the maximum number of examples of methods and systems in which client information gathered is retained, the records made and kept in large institutions or organisations, e.g. hospitals, will be emphasised but the principles of information gathering and recording can be applied to all workplaces, it is a matter scale to meet need of a particular location.

The rules of confidentiality are the same whatever the source of information or the method by which it is recorded. This includes records held in GP practices, nursing homes and residential homes, as well as in hospitals. It is important to remember that the client has an absolute right to expect that the information disclosed to a health care professional is treated in confidence, obtained in a tactful and sympathetic manner, and acknowledges the respect and dignity due to the individual at all times (see Chapter 2).

Key words: Confidentiality; computer; information; password; medical records; library; manual records (case notes); electronic; client master index; log out; log in; data; Data Protection Act; Caldicott Report

Confidentiality

As a carer, you will be responsible for maintaining at all times your employer's policy on confidentiality. You should therefore ask to see a copy of the policy to ensure that you, and others, observe the rules. The policy will cover many aspects of your work, including disclosure of information to internal and external sources and use of electronic computer systems.

Familiarity with the policy on confidentiality will ensure that you never unintentionally breach it, which may not only cause distress to the client and their family, but can also carry severe penalties for the person who breaches the policy. The relationship between the client and health care professional is based entirely on trust and it is essential to both the physical and mental well-being of clients that this trust is guaranteed by strict observance of the confidentiality rules.

A few of the commonest ways in which confidentiality can be breached are listed below:

- Medical records (case notes) left in an unattended area
- Failure to establish whether information may be disclosed and establishing the identity of the requester
- Failure to log out of computer systems, allowing others access through your password, to information to which they may not be entitled
- A visual display unit or computer monitor (VDU), which is inappropriately sited, so that the screen with client information is visible to non-health care professionals
- Allowing your password to be known and used by other members of staff.
- Conducting conversations (including on the telephone) in an area where the conversation may be overheard by members of the public, e.g. in an outpatient clinic or any public area

Every member of staff is responsible for client confidentiality in accordance with their employer's policy and any breaches, either by yourself or by others, should be reported immediately to a senior member of staff.

Confidentiality and computer systems

Access levels

Access levels are a means of controlling which users have access to various modules on the computer system. You will be given a password appropriate to your needs for carrying out your duties. For example, you may need to access the bed states function, but not the out-patients appointment system. You may also need to be able to input, amend or delete information on some functions, but on others you will be granted access on a read-only basis. The password you are given will therefore reflect your need to undertake your duties.

It is essential that you never divulge your password to another person and that when you have finished using the computer system, you log out before leaving the terminal. This will prevent anyone else accessing the system using your password.

Siting of terminals

Terminals must always be sited with the screens facing away from public areas, so that the information is only visible to the user. Never walk away from the terminal leaving information on the screen and always log out of the system, however short your absence, and log in again to the system on your return.

Confidentiality and medical records libraries

As the library is an area containing highly confidential information in the form of manual medical records (case notes) access to the library is usually strictly controlled. If you are not allowed access to the library to retrieve case notes, the medical records library staff will be available to retrieve them for you and, if required, print hard copies of medical records held on microfilm.

Data Protection Act 1998

This Act[2] came into effect in the UK in March 2000 and gives clients/patients and/or their legal representatives the right to apply for access to their manual and computer medical records. This Act applies only to the medical records of living clients.

The eight principles of data protection

(1) Personal data shall be processed fairly and lawfully and, in particular, shall not be processed unless:
 (a) at least one of the conditions in Schedule 2 is met, and
 (b) in the case of sensitive personal data, at least one of the conditions in Schedule 3 is also met.

 NB: Schedule 2 covers the rights of data subjects and others, and Schedule 3 covers conditions of notification by data controllers.
(2) Personal data shall be obtained only for one or more specified and lawful purposes, and shall not further be processed in any manner incompatible with that purpose or those purposes.
(3) Personal data shall be adequate, relevant and not excessive in relation to the purpose or purposes for which they are processed.
(4) Personal data shall be accurate and where necessary, kept up to date.
(5) Personal data processed for any purpose or purposes shall not be kept for longer than is necessary for that purpose or those purposes.
(6) Personal data shall be processed in accordance with the rights of data subjects under this act.
(7) Appropriate technical and organisational measures shall be taken against unauthorised or unlawful processing of personal data and against accidental loss or destruction of, or damage to, personal data.
(8) Personal data shall not be transferred to a country or territory outside the European Economic Area unless that country or territory ensures an

adequate level of protection for the rights and freedoms of data subjects in relation to the processing of personal data.

There are strict guidelines for dealing with requests made under the Data Protection Act 1998. Requests must be submitted in writing and an application for access form completed, on which the requester's signature must be authorised by a person with professional status, e.g. a minister of religion or a school teacher.

Requests for access to medical records in a hospital are usually processed by the medical records department, which will obtain the authority of the consultant who treated the patient/client, to release the records to the requester. There is usually a small administrative fee charged for processing the request.

It is important to remember that the guidelines for requesting access to medical records also apply to clients during an in-patient episode, and that the request should be referred to the medical records department. Patients should not be given informal access to their medical records whilst on the ward, but their request should be passed to the appropriate department for processing.

Access to Health Records Act 1990

This Act[3] applies to the medical records of deceased clients. The guidelines are similar to those for requests made under the Data Protection Act 1998 in that requests for access must be submitted in writing and the authority of the appropriate consultant obtained, prior to release of the records to the requester.

If you receive enquiries relating to access to the medical records of a deceased client, either refer the request to your immediate manager or to the medical records department. This will ensure that the request is dealt with according to the guidelines and that you do not become involved with inappropriate disclosure of information or breaches of client confidentiality.

Medical records libraries

Current medical records (case notes)

In hospitals the manual medical records (case notes) are stored and filed numerically in the medical records library. Every client who has an in-patient or out-patient episode is registered on the 'Patient Master Index' and allocated a unique hospital number. This number is often computer-generated, although if it is not, and a manual system is still in place, it must be entered on the computer system against the client's name and details. A computer-printed label should be affixed to the front cover of the case notes folder and the client's name also written in black ink on the front cover. Case notes will be filed in the library by hospital number, not by name.

On each occasion that the client attends an out-patient clinic or is admitted to a ward, the case notes will be required by the clinicians treating the client and will be retrieved from the library for that purpose. When that episode is complete, the case notes are returned to the library for storage, until they are required again.

Archived medical records (case notes)

Because libraries do not have a limitless capacity for the storage of medical records, it is usual to microfilm the records of clients who have not attended the hospital for a certain period of time. This procedure releases space for the records of current clients to be filed in the medical records library.

The film spools on which the information from the paper records is held are similar to the ones used in cameras. It is very easy to obtain hard (paper) copies from the film, by feeding the film through a printing machine, identifying the documents required and then printing copies. Once the medical records have been microfilmed and the film has undergone a quality check, the case notes are destroyed in accordance with security and confidentiality procedures.

Although microfilming remains the most commonly used method for storage of old records, during recent years laser disks and CDs have become increasingly popular for storage purposes.

Each hospital will have its own retention and destruction policy for its medical records, taking into account the minimum retention periods recommended by the Department of Health; other reasons can force retention such as research projects, medico-legal issues and medical audit.

Movement of case notes

The medical record is essential to client care and must be available to health care professionals at all times. A record must therefore always be kept of the current location of case notes, so that they can be retrieved when required, particularly for emergency admissions.

Tracer cards

Tracer cards are used in manual storage systems as a means of recording the current location of a set of case notes. When case notes are retrieved from the library, a tracer card must be completed and placed in the space left by the removal of the case notes. The tracer card will state the date on which the file was retrieved, the name of the clinic or ward to which the case notes were despatched and the name of the person who requested the case notes. This information allows anyone else requiring the case notes to identify their current location.

Case notes, which are in circulation around the hospital, may be moved between departments, prior to being returned to the library for storage. Every department, ward and office, should therefore maintain a log book in which the movements of case notes are recorded, similar to the tracer card held in the library, so that there is an efficient system of identifying whether or not case notes are currently in the department.

Electronic case note tracking systems

The use of tracer cards and log books to record the movements of case notes is increasingly being superseded by electronic tracking systems. The advantage of an electronic tracking system is that the current location of case notes can be viewed by any user with access to a computer terminal, whereas tracer cards can only be accessed by medical records staff in the library.

Obtaining case notes from other hospitals

When you need to obtain medical records from another hospital, it is usual for such requests to be made through the medical records library. The library will contact the hospital concerned and arrange for the transfer of the records by the fastest and safest route. As this process can take a few days, except in case of emergencies, the request should be made as far in advance as possible of the date on which the records are required.

Obtaining client information

There are many sources from which information relating to the client can be obtained, which will need to be recorded in the individual record to ensure that it is complete, with all details up to date and accurate. The main sources of information are listed below:

- General practitioner (GP) or tertiary referral letter
- Client pre-registration questionnaire, which is usually sent to the client with the first out-patient appointment letter
- Direct from the client at an out-patient clinic attendance
- Information already in the client's case notes
- Information held by the admissions office (for in-patients)
- Direct from the client, or their relatives, during an in-patient episode
- Colleagues who may have been involved in the care of the client
- Hospital patient administration computer systems
- Personal record systems of nursing/residential homes

The main methods of obtaining information fall into three categories:

- Face-to-face interviews
- By telephone
- Written information

Face-to-face interviews

This method allows you to obtain details direct from the client and/or their relatives or carer. It provides the opportunity to raise any queries about the accuracy of the information and to confirm that details are complete and correct.

Always begin the interview by introducing yourself, ensuring that your name badge is clearly visible, and explain the purpose of the interview.

It is sometimes necessary to ask a client for information of a sensitive nature which may give rise to some distress and embarrassment. However, if you have explained the reason why the information is required at the outset and asked the questions in a sensitive manner, the client will usually respond favourably, enabling you to complete the details in the record.

Face-to-face interviews should always be conducted in a sensitive and tactful manner, in a quiet area where the conversation cannot be overheard, and with regard to the client's right to respect, privacy and dignity.

Written information

Written information should be legible, accurate and concise. A brief heading identifying the subject contained in the message immediately informs the reader of the type of information being conveyed. For example, if the heading reads 'Urology Clinic – Booking of Appointments', the writer has in just five words identified which clinic is being referred to and the activity within that clinic.

Written information should always include the names of the sender and intended recipient, the date, the time (when a message is received by telephone and written down), the department or location and, if appropriate, the telephone number of the caller. These details enable the sender and recipient to contact each other without delay, should the need arise. In cases where the written information refers to a specific client, in addition to the full name add the client's unique identification (ID) number and the date of birth. This ensures that clients with the same or similar surnames are not confused, which can result in serious consequences. Where unusual names or messages are being taken, the spellings should be ascertained in order that mistakes are avoided. Illegibly written information can be very dangerous and have a detrimental effect upon care. If there is even the slightest doubt about the legibility of hand-written information, for example, on a nursing record or prescription sheet, always check for accuracy prior to taking any action.

Telephone

This is a commonly used method of obtaining and exchanging information but is also one where misunderstandings and errors can easily occur. Many of these errors are caused by the speakers failing to communicate in an articulate manner, which in turn can lead to confusion and misunderstanding.

The following guidelines will help you to avoid the common pitfalls of obtaining information through use of the telephone.

- Identify yourself when making or receiving a telephone call.
- Confirm you have the correct department or location.
- State briefly the reason for the call, for example: 'This is the admissions office with a query on your bed state.'
- Deliver the message as concisely as possible and, if appropriate, in the correct sequence of events.

- Ask the person to whom you are speaking to repeat back to you any details you feel might need confirmation, for example: 'There are eight empty beds on the ward at present.'
- Make a brief written record of the conversation, including the name of the person to whom you spoke, the date and time of the call and what action, if any, was agreed and taken as a result.

Receiving and transmitting information

Facsimile transmissions (fax)

Information may also be sent or received by use of facsimile transmissions. Extreme care needs to be taken in using this method of exchanging information and wherever possible, transmissions should only be made to a facsimile number which is classified as a 'safe haven'.

All transmissions should include a front (cover) sheet on your hospital or workplace official headed paper, showing a statement relating to the confidentiality of the information being transmitted, in case the transmission is misrouted.

Requests for a client's information to be faxed should be made in writing, on official headed paper, showing a contact name and telephone number. Verbal requests for information to be faxed should not be accepted.

Authority to fax a client's information to a requester should be obtained from the appropriate manager, before the transmission is undertaken because it is not always a suitable mode of transfer.

Electronic mail (e-mail)

Electronic mail is an extremely fast method of receiving and sending information. However, because of the ease with which e-mail exchanges can occur, the rules relating to confidentiality are unfortunately not always as strictly observed as with other forms of communication.

Today most institutions have an external e-mail system (internet) and larger ones have internal e-mail systems, with access to both systems by passwords. When transmitting a client's information by electronic mail, it is essential to apply the same rules on confidentiality as for other methods of receiving and sending sensitive client data.

Computer systems

Information about clients is increasingly being held on computer systems, as well as in paper records (case notes). Many health care professionals and administrative and clerical staff contribute to the inputting and updating of client information, all of whom have responsibility for ensuring that the information on the record is accurate and up to date.

To access the various functions on the computer system, you will be allocated a password, which will allow you a level of access to undertake your duties. Some of the functions will only allow you to read information, whilst others will allow you to input and update information. The allocation of passwords is usually dependent upon satisfactory completion of training in the required computer systems.

Information is increasingly becoming available electronically, including test results and digitised images from radiology departments, so that paper results and radiographic films are gradually becoming obsolete. The main advantage of this move from paper to electronic records is that information is quickly available to all users 24 hours a day 365 days a year, whereas paper records may be difficult to obtain if required outside working hours of administrative and clerical staff.

Recording client information

Manual records (case notes)

Although information is increasingly available electronically, paper medical records (case notes) are still extremely important and non-availability of the case notes may result in the cancellation of appointments, admissions, treatments and care.

Entering information in the client's record requires legible handwriting, preferably using a pen with black ink and in addition to medical terminology, the use of good, basic English. This prevents any confusion arising from misinterpretation of illegible handwriting or misunderstanding of unfamiliar or ambiguous words. All entries in the medical record must be dated and signed by the writer, with a legible signature.

The case notes folder containing the medical records may include a number of dividers with printed instructions on which documentation should be filed in each section. There will also be mount sheets on which test results should be affixed in the correct order. All documentation should be secured within the case notes folder to ensure that it does not become detached from the record and irretrievably lost.

A neat case notes folder with the contents filed in the correct section and all documentation secured facilitates the extraction of information from the case notes to the benefit of all users.

Inputting on computer systems

The data which you input on the computer system will be accessed by many other members of staff and it is therefore essential that you check the accuracy of the information, before inputting on the system. (See the Eight Principles of the Data Protection Act 1998 above).

Many of the individual's demographic details, such as their address, will have been input at the time of registration and will require amending, if for example, the client has changed their address. At the same time telephone numbers and GP details can be checked and updated as necessary.

To ensure that the requirement of the Data Protection Act 1998 that personal data are kept up to date is met, clients should be asked at each out-patient attendance or in-patient episode whether there are any changes in their demographic details.

Patient administration system

Every hospital has a patient administration system of which the patient master index is the foundation. It is essential that the information on the index is always accurate and up to date, as other modules within the system extract demographic details from it.

The index consists of the following:

- Hospital number
- Client's surname
- Client's forename(s)
- Title
- Date of birth
- Address (including postcode)
- Marital status
- General practitioner
- Sex

Although considerably more information of clients' details is held on the computer system, the above data should be input at the time a client is registered on the patient administration system and allocated a hospital number.

Further clients' details are obtained usually through the use of a questionnaire, which is sent to clients with their first out-patient appointment and returned to the hospital in advance of the clinic date. These details can then be input on the patient administration system and confirmed with the client at the time of their attendance at clinic. In the event of an emergency admission, the relevant information should either be obtained direct from the client or their relatives.

Failure to keep information accurate and up to date can have serious consequences, such as not being able to contact a client quickly if a test result indicates that an urgent clinic attendance is required or a client may miss the opportunity for admission when a bed becomes available at short notice but cannot be contacted by telephone.

Other locations where clients receive care will have similar formal record systems and many are now computerised so that the information in this section is very relevant to them.

Menu

The menu lists all the functions available on the module. Against each function listed there will be a code, which when entered will give you access to the information, provided your password allows you entry.

Help facility

The patient administration system provides a help facility to assist in completing the fields shown on the screen, particularly the mandatory fields. If you request help against a field, e.g. religion, the screen will display a list of options (usually referred to as the drop-down list) from which you can select the appropriate religion and add it to the client's record.

The Caldicott report 1997

Ensuring security and confidentiality in the NHS

A key recommendation of the Caldicott Report[4] was the establishment of Caldicott Guardians throughout the National Health Service (NHS) with responsibility for the confidentiality and security of clients' information.

The Caldicott Guardian is usually a senior health care professional, with wide-ranging responsibilities which include the way in which data are obtained, why it is required, how it is used and flows of information which contain client-identifiable data.

The ease with which electronic information can be accessed and exchanged has necessitated the need for strict security of both manual and computer systems, to ensure that the eight principles of the Data Protection Act 1998 are maintained at all times.

Both the Caldicott Report 1997 and the Data Protection Act 1998 are relevant to the work undertaken by all health care professionals, and although detailed knowledge is not necessary, a broad understanding of the Report and the Act are essential, to avoid any breaches of confidentiality occurring.

Summary

Information concerning clients may be held either in manual records (case notes) or on computer systems. As a health care professional, you will have responsibility for obtaining, inputting, updating and retrieving confidential and sensitive information.

In both manual and computer systems it is essential that the information is accurate and up to date, which is as important for recording the client's telephone number as it is for clinical details.

When not in current use, case notes must be stored in the medical records library or appropriate secure location and case notes must never be left in unsupervised areas in clinics or on wards or in public areas.

Computer terminals must never be sited where the screens are visible to the public and should never be left unattended with information showing on the screen. Always log out of the system on completion of accessing the information required and never allow your password to be known or used by others.

Confidentiality of information applies equally to manual and electronic records in accordance with the Caldicott Report 1997 and the Data Protection Act

1998. Familiarity with the policies relating to confidentiality will ensure that you never breach the policies, for which there can be severe penalties.

The relationship between the client and health care professional is based entirely on trust and it is essential to both the physical and mental well-being of the client, that this trust is guaranteed by strict observance of the rules relating to client confidentiality.

References

1. Royal College of Nursing (2004) *RCN Guidance on Professional Matters for Health Cave Assistants and Nurse Cadets*. Royal College of Nursing, London.
2. Department of Health (1998) *Data Protection Act 1998*. Department of Health, London.
3. Department of Health (1990) *Access to Health Records Act 1990*. Department of Health, London.
4. Department of Health (1997) *Caldicott Report*. Department of Health, London.

Further reading

Organisational policies and procedures relating to confidentiality of patient records.

Chapter 7
Basic biomechanics: movement and handling equipment

Fay Reid

Overview

We all need to move. We move to find, prepare and eat food. We move to get away from danger. We wriggle and fidget to make ourselves comfortable, to even out the pressures when we are lying, sitting or standing. There are some people who, because of disease, frailty or trauma, cannot move themselves, so that there is very little care that is undertaken for, or with, a client that does not involve moving them.

When you assist clients with their daily activities it is essential that you know what you are doing and the result of your actions, otherwise you could injure the client or yourself. The task of moving people is a complex one as they are almost always longer, heavier or larger than you think. Human beings respond to gravity. They will fall over if, because of illness or injury, they cannot weight-bear, or control their balance or musculo-skeletal system. Clients do not have handles, or grab-slots, they can be stiffer or floppier than you imagine, have arms and legs that wave about and do not always do what they should, or stay where you have placed them. They have a large, almost central hinge and if an upward pressure is exerted on either side of it, once it is off a supportive surface it will fold. People can be physically unstable, forgetful of instructions and behave in an irrational and unpredictable manner.

To help each client move as normally as possible requires knowledge of normal patterns of movement; how disease can alter these; the methods to enable them to use the ability that remains; and knowledge of, and competence in, the use of handling techniques and equipment. To gain knowledge and develop these skills you need to watch demonstrations by expert practitioners and then practise for yourself, under the supervision of a skilled and competent practitioner. Very few people learn to drive a car safely or play a musical instrument by reading a book or without practice. Accidents happen because of the unexpected.

The aim of Chapters 7 and 8 is to help you avoid the unexpected and reinforce what you have been told and shown. These chapters include information on the legislation, normal patterns of movement, causes and effects of cumulative strain, the commoner types of equipment, the content of mobility, risk and task assessment, and the analysis of some common tasks. They will not describe manual handling techniques, as these need to be learnt under supervision following demonstration and practice. As it is easier to learn by doing, activities are included to encourage you to reflect on your own patterns of movement and the application of this knowledge when you are helping others to move.

Key words: Legal responsibilities; effect of gravity; patterns of movement; static muscle work; care plan; client mobility; environment; task and risk assessments; environment; equipment; safe systems; team lifting; synchronisation

Legislation to prevent work-related injury

It has been known since at least 1965, that people who give physical care to others can be injured by the work they do. There has been legislation since 1974 to reduce the risk of work-related injury. The umbrella act is the Health and Safety at Work Act (HASWA) 1974, which contains responsibilities for your employer and you, the employee[1]. The main duties for employers are stated in Chapter 37, Part 1, section 2, sub-sections (a) to (e). Your **employer** has, so far as is reasonable, a statutory duty to:

- Provide and maintain equipment and safe systems of work that are safe and without risks to health
- Ensure safety and absence of risks to health in connection with use, handling, storage and transport of articles and substances
- Provide information, instruction, training and supervision as necessary, to ensure the health and safety of employees at work
- Maintain the place of work in a safe condition without risks to health and provide and maintain means of access to and egress from it that are safe and without such risks
- Provide and maintain a working environment for employers that is safe, without risks to health, and adequate as regards facilites and arrangements for their employees at work

Section 7 outlines the duties of **employees** to:

- Take reasonable care of the health and safety of themselves and of other people affected by their acts or omissions at work
- Co-operate with the employer to ensure their own and other people's safety at all times
- Use equipment which is provided, safely
- Take the opportunities that they are given, in relation to training, instruction and supervision

Employees have a common law duty of care. This means they must exercise 'reasonable skill and care' in their relationship with their employer or their colleagues. In addition they must take reasonable care of themselves and other people at work. They should maintain their own health and fitness to do the job and also, where necessary, wear protective clothing/work attire designed to enable them to carry out all aspects of their work safely. This includes clothing and footwear provided by the employer enabling them to lift and move clients safely; protective garments – aprons, overalls, and where appropriate, gloves which prevent contamination and infection (see Chapters 9, 10 and 11).

HASWA is a general Act which covers all employed and self-employed people so does not go into detail about specific hazardous activities or occupations which are known to have a foreseeable risk of ill health or injury. In June 1990, the European Council accepted a directive that addressed specific known health and safety risks at work. Governments that signed the directive had until 1 January 1993 to comply with it. The following regulations were tabled in November 1992 and came into effect on 1 January 1993.

Management of the Health and Safety at Work Regulations (MHSWR) 1992

The MHSWR require the employer to carry out a risk assessment if the work that is undertaken by employees is likely to give rise to injury or illness. Guidance on these regulations was published in 1992 and updated in 1998[2].

Manual Handling Operations Regulations (MHOR) 1992

MHOR place a statutory duty on the employer to undertake an assessment of the load, the task, environment and the individual staff member's capability to undertake the task if there is any risk of injury in the load handling task. Manual handling is defined in the regulations as 'transporting or supporting of a load (including the lifting, putting down, pushing, pulling carrying or moving thereof) by hand or bodily force'[3]. The load must be a 'discrete movable object' and includes a 'human client'. The Health and Safety Executive published guidance on the regulations in 1992 with a second edition in 1998[4]. The Health Service Advisory Committee published guidance on manual handling of loads in the health services in 1992, which is specific to the care services[5].

Provision and Use of Work Equipment Regulations (PUWER) 1992

PUWER was up-dated in 1998[6]. These make explicit the requirement in sub-section 2a of HASWA for the provision and maintenance of equipment and systems of work that are, as far as is reasonably practicable, safe. Work equipment is defined as 'any machinery, appliance, apparatus, tool or installation for use at work, (whether exclusively or not)'. Regulation 4 says 'Every employer shall ensure that work equipment is so constructed or adapted as to be suitable for the purpose for which it is used or provided.'

Lifting Operations and Lifting Equipment Regulations (LOLER) 1998

Regulation 4 of LOLER requires an employer to ensure that lifting equipment has sufficient strength and stability for each load and Regulation 5 that anyone using (in or on) the equipment will not be crushed, trapped or struck, or fall from the carrier. Although these regulations apply in the main to industry they are applicable to lifting people. The Health and Safety Executive (HSE) published guidance on MHOR[4] and an approved code of practice for the MHSWR in 1992 and 1998[2]. The Health Service Advisory Committee (HSAC) published guidance on manual handling that was specific to the care services in 1982, 1992 and 1998. It is not possible to cover this guidance to the legislation in detail here. The references at the end of the chapter gives you sources of more information.

Activity 7.1

Try to read the guidance to the MHOR and MHSWR. Make yourself familiar with your local policies and guidelines concerning safe manual handling. These should be available in your workplace and are based on the Health and Safety at Work etc. Act 1974.

Normal patterns of movement

Body shape

Figure 7.1 illustrates the shape of the body. The body is shaped like a well-filled ice cream cone. The weight of the head, neck, upper limbs and trunk, from hip joint upward, is approximately 68% of total body weight. It is supported by two lower limbs weighing about 15.7% of body weight each and forming approximately 50% of total height. The base, that is the feet, supporting this structure, is around 15% of its height. This shape is innately unstable. It is like placing a large, top-heavy bouquet of flowers in a triangular shaped vase where the base of the vase is the narrowest part.

Activity 7.2

Stand, with your feet together, in front of a full-length mirror. What do you see? Consider the width of your feet to be about 20 cm (8 inches) then work upwards to the maximum width at the top of the thighs which may be about 35–40 cm. Feel the bony pelvis which forms the cup of the 'ice-cream cone'. From the waist to the shoulders the trunk remains more or less the same width. Emerging from the shoulders there is the narrow column of the neck that supports the head, which weighs approximately 5 kg. Is this a stable, rectangular shape, or something that resembles a triangle balanced on its point, topped by a rectangle supporting a sphere balanced on a thin column?

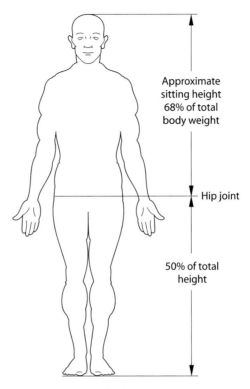

Approximate
sitting height
68% of total
body weight

Hip joint

50% of total
height

Fig. 7.1 Diagram showing the shape of the body.

Spinal curves

Figure 7.2. illustrates the spinal curves. The shape of a human being makes them fundamentally unstable in an upright position and in order to maintain an upright position they have to be able to defy gravity. Gravity is always there and if we lose consciousness for whatever reason we will fall over. When a baby is born he or she is totally floppy and unable to support any part of her or himself. The spine is basically C-shaped and before the baby can sit he or she has to be able to support their own head. Once that has been achieved the baby then starts to roll over and push him- or herself up on hands and arms until they can crawl and sit. The baby will need to have sitting balance before he or she can stand. This early activity develops the spine from its original C-shape to an inward curve at the neck and a further inward curve at the lower back. It is these curves that we need to maintain when sitting, standing or leaning forward.

Dynamic and static muscle work

Normal movement requires muscle work. Muscles shorten to flex a joint and lengthen to take it back to its resting position. Contraction of the muscle is followed by relaxation, flexion by extension. When muscles contract the blood flow is restricted due to pressure within the muscle. Blood flows back as the muscle relaxes. In this way the muscle acts as a pump to ensure that the muscle is

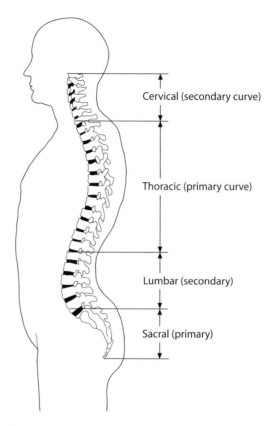

Fig. 7.2   The spinal curves.

supplied with the blood it needs. This is dynamic muscle work and this type of work can continue for a long time provided the rate and rhythm is suitable.

In static work the muscle is held in a compressed state for a period of time and this most frequently happens when we hold a forward leaning posture, such as leaning across a client to support them when they are lying on their side near the edge of a bed. In this forward leaning position the muscles of the back and legs are involved in static muscle work to hold us up and stop us falling as the trunk is held beyond the body's centre of gravity.

Many of the tasks that are undertaken when assisting people to carry out the activities of daily living involve both dynamic and static muscle work and it is the static effort that contributes most to any fatigue or pain that we may feel.

Activity 7.3

Clench your hand to make a fist and keep it clenched for at least a minute. Consider how your fingers feel when you open your fist. During the period the hand was clenched blood flow into your hand and fingers was reduced and in addition the waste products could not be removed. What you are feeling in the muscles of the fingers is a mixture of the accumulation of waste products because the venous return was reduced, arterial blood returning to the fingers blood and the fatigue of static muscle work.

Effect of tension and anxiety

When assisting clients, or at home, try to avoid being tense when you work. Tension and anxiety can affect your muscles and increase fatigue levels. Take a tip from weight lifters and if you have to support, push, pull, lift or lower do not hold your breath and remember to breathe out at the time of maximum exertion. Holding your breath increases intra-abdominal pressure and also blood pressure. If you have been taught to control the deepest abdominal muscle, transversus abdominis, engage it, to help brace your spine when manual handling. In addition tension and anxiety are easily transmitted to the client through your hands. This may cause them to lose confidence in your ability to move them safely and comfortably which, in turn, may make them tense and more difficult to handle.

Sitting, standing, and walking

Sitting, standing and walking are activities that the majority of people have been able to do for as long as they can remember; because each action is taken without needing to think about it, it is all taken for granted. Before you help others to carry out these activities you need to consider these movements in detail and work out what has to happen before we can stand, sit or walk so that this knowledge can be applied to assist clients with any difficulties with mobility they may have.

Standing

When clients have had a stroke the physiotherapist will test them for trunk stability before they start to stand them. Do not attempt to manually transfer a client, from bed to chair, or stand them, if they do not have sitting balance. Without trunk stability we will fall when sitting or standing.

Sitting

The human body is more stable when it is sitting upright; however sitting should also carry a health warning. We find it difficult to maintain our spinal curves

---

Activity 7.4

(1) Sit, without leaning forwards or backwards, on a chair with a firm seat and place your hands under your buttocks. As you sit upright you should be able to feel the bony projections (ischial tuberosities) you are sitting on. The weight of the upper body will make it difficult to remove your hands from under you.
(2) Now move forwards so that your nose is above your toes.
(3) Then lean backwards against the chair. Think what happens to the weight distribution on your hands each time you move.
(4) Finally, fold your arms in front of you and stand up from each of the three positions, leaning back against the chair, nose over toes, or sitting upright, without using your hands and arms to help. Which of the three positions is the easiest? When you are standing from a sitting position think what the muscles of the thighs have to do.

with unsupported sitting and if we are working at a desk or table with a flat top we end up with our spine in a C-shaped curve, which puts it under strain. In order to be able to assist someone to stand from a sitting position we need to consider how we alter the weight distribution of our trunk as we prepare to stand.

Walking

The majority of people do not remember learning to walk so we do not think of the movements involved when walking. Disease processes often alter the way people can walk so rehabilitation for people who have developed difficulties when walking may involve encouraging and teaching people to walk with as normal a way of walking (gait) as possible. Normal gait involves balancing and weight bearing on one leg while swinging the other leg in front of the one being stood on. The next activity is to think what happens to the body when we walk.

Activity 7.5

Stand with feet together and think whether you feel steady or not. Now stand on one foot. Can you maintain your balance? While standing on one foot close your eyes. Is it still as easy to balance? You may find that you wobble a bit or find that it is quite difficult. The reason is that we need both eyes and sense of balance to maintain our upright position. If the sense of balance is lost the eyes can help to keep us in the upright position. Open your eyes. Place your hands on your hips and take some steps forward. What is happening to your legs and weight as you do so? Although you may find it more difficult to walk slowly like this, you will notice that your hips and weight move until your weight is over the supporting leg. In order for clients to be able to walk without support they need to be able to stand, balance, take their body weight onto another position and balance each leg in turn.

Before you start to stand or walk a client it is important that you know if the client can do this and how far this activity can be sustained. There is no point in trying to walk a client to a chair in the day room 10 m away if the client can only walk 2 m.

Use of body weight

The classic principles of lifting state that the strong leg and thigh muscles should be used to power a lift, but that is not always possible. It can really only apply to a vertical lift, where the load is below knuckle height and can be held close. These principles do not cover such activities as pushing and pulling when standing on the far side of a trolley or bed, or the horizontal movement in 'moving someone up the bed'. The client is seldom close to you and the human load may be as heavy or heavier than you are. Unless you have weight lifted or trained, the muscles of the upper body and arms are neither strong nor powerful. The shoulder joint has the distinction of being the most mobile in the body. The head of the humerus fits into a shallow cavity and the joint capsule is very loose. Several muscle tendons help to stabilise the joint but the humerus can be dislocated fairly easily from its socket. If your elbows move away from your body as they flex when pulling something towards you, you are using arms and shoulders to power the movement, not body weight.

In order to use body weight you must be able to move your weight from side to side or backwards and forwards in whichever direction you want to exert the force, so your feet must be apart. Hip distance is insufficient to move body weight from side to side; forward and backward weight transfer requires one foot to be a good walking stride in front of the other. Tennis players, on the base line, waiting to receive service from their opponents are a good example of transferring weight from side to side. They need to be able to move quickly in either direction but be sufficiently stable to return the service with power should it land anywhere near them.

Activity 7.6

Do this activity in front of a full-length mirror, if possible, and then you can see just how much you can move. Face the mirror and place your feet about hip distance apart so that ankles and knees are in line with your hips. Keeping both feet on the ground take your weight onto one foot and then transfer it across to the other. How far did you move? Did you almost over balance? Now place your feet at least twice that distance apart and repeat the side-to-side movement. Now stand with one foot in front of the other and try transferring your weight from front to back and back again. How far could you move? Take a good walking stride forward and repeat the weight transfer. It may seem strange standing with feet more than hip distance apart but you will be more stable, it is far more effective and it will reduce the risk of injury to your arms, shoulders and back.

Equipment

Familiarise yourself with the client-handling equipment and make friends with it so that you are competent and confident when using it. It has been provided to help you help clients move as safely and comfortably as possible for both of you. To acquire a painful back because you moved a client who was too heavy for you is not helpful for you, your client or your colleagues.

Beds

Hospitals have used King's Fund style beds for many years and they remain the standard bed in a large number of hospitals. They all have height adjustable mattress platforms, though the mechanism for raising the mattress platform varies. They all have the ability to tilt at either end and therefore raise either the head end or the foot end, (this is known as the Trendelenburg position), between 5 and 7 degrees with a maximum of 12 degrees depending on the height of the mattress platform. All models have an adjustable back support though it varies from being angled forward from the bed head or part of the mattress platform that can be raised. The angle of the back support is approximately 60 degrees. It is essentially a sitting up bed, but clients slip towards the foot of the bed when reclining at 60 degrees due to the weight distribution of the human body and the effect of gravity. To prevent this the tilt mechanism can be used. By raising the foot of the mattress platform 5 degrees or so the client cannot slip up the incline.

The difficulty for staff when caring for clients in King's Fund beds is that the weight of the client, mattress and mattress platform has to be raised by the physical effort of one member of staff. If a wind-up bed is being used the handle is low down on the frame and staff may have to kneel or stoop to operate it. In addition they are winding upwards the total weight of mattress platform and everything it supports using the relatively weak muscles of arms and shoulders. With foot-operated pedals care workers are using the power in one leg to raise the combined weight while balancing on the other. In many instances these beds are not routinely maintained and many of them go up and down in a series of jerks.

The weight limit for these beds is usually about 180 kg. This limit is often indicated on the frame of the mattress platform. If it is exceeded, while the bed will seldom break, the raising and lowering mechanism can be affected. Some designs will tip if too much weight is put on the head end. The average weight of a British woman aged between 18 and 65 years is 62.5 kg (about 9 stone 12 pounds). If there is a 62.5 kg client sitting in the bed and two, average weight, care workers are positioned with a knee on the bed at the head end of the bed, prior to sliding her up the bed, all the weight is on the top half of the bed and it adds up to 187.5 kg. Hospitals are beginning to phase out these older beds and replacing them with electrically operated variable posture beds, sometimes referred to as 'profiling beds'.

Electrically operated variable posture beds

Some hospitals have already replaced their King's Fund beds with electrically operated variable posture beds (Fig. 7.3) and others are planning to do so. Since 1990 an increasing number and variety of these beds are available with mattress platforms that are in three or four sections. These can be adjusted to a more chair-like position and the hinge at knee level can be raised to allow a supported, bent knee position which again would help to keep the client in place. These provide a more stable base than a tilted King's Fund bed. The variable posture bed allows clients some control over their position in bed and lessens the workload of the nursing staff.

Fixed height beds

No person dependent on care workers for assistance with most of the activities of daily living, should be cared for in a fixed height bed. However, many care staff working in the community are faced with that situation. The bed is usually a domestic divan that may be single or double. Care given to any person in these

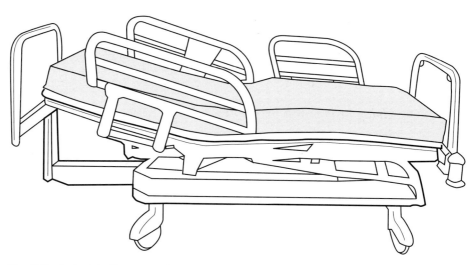

Fig. 7.3 A electrically operated variable posture bed.

beds is highly likely to cause cumulative postural strain through the static muscle work caused by the stoop and or stretch to reach the person in the bed. The double divan makes giving care even more hazardous. Kneeling by a divan bed is not necessarily going to reduce the risk of injury. Some caring activities require the care worker to stand. In addition not every one can kneel comfortably for a period of time. You also need to remember that domestic beds are not necessarily in good condition and may not contribute to assisting the person in it or improving the independence of the person in it. Kneeling on the bed to get near to the client is not always safe.

Height-adjustable, variable posture beds can be obtained, usually following an assessment of the dependency of the client, though they may not always be available immediately. As a temporary measure the bed can be raised by the use of extension legs, blocks, but only those designed for the purpose. Paint tins are not an acceptable substitute. If beds need to be moved castors can be provided, including castors with brakes. As with all beds, you need to remember that if you have to move the bed to reach the client, the effort involved is that of pushing or pulling the weight of the bed plus the weight of the client against the resistance of the floor covering. Another aspect to think about is that the client may be able to get out of bed once it is raised but not necessarily get back in again. They should not be manually lifted on to the bed. The other problem with a fixed raised bed is that should the client fall, or try to get out of bed when there is no one nearby to assist him or her, any resulting injury may be in direct proportion to the distance fallen.

Special beds

These are fluidised, stand up and turning beds, low air loss and water beds. They are usually hired to meet a client's specific problems. It is beyond the remit of this chapter to discuss the many varieties of special beds and mattresses available. You need to ensure that you have been shown how to operate these beds and you have practised with the bed provided and read carefully the instructions and the manufacturer's literature.

Using beds – first principles

The bed should be at the highest level convenient for the people working with the client, but at the lowest level when the client is on their own. Clients do fall out of bed. If they fall from a bed with its mattress platform 800–900 mm high, their injuries are likely to be far greater than if they fall from one where the mattress platform is 350–450 mm high. With the bed at its lowest level it is possible for the average-sized client to put their hands on the floor to support themselves. If feet and legs go first then there is a chance that the feet may reach the floor first and help to support them.

Side rails

Beds are occasionally fitted with side rails, particularly if the client is a child or is restless. Be very careful with the use of side rails as both clients and staff can be injured. Their use should only follow careful risk assessment and discussion with the client and their relatives. There are two types, folding and split and some beds are supplied with side rails already in position. They can often be old, poorly maintained or incompatible with the bed on which they are being used. Four hazard notices about side rails have been issued by the Medical Devices Directorate since 1997. They cite the risk of falls, entrapment or asphyxiation either due to clamp-on-sides moving away from the bed, side rails that are incompatible, or in poor condition. Not only can clients be injured or die from asphyxiation but also staff trying to free clients can be injured as well.

Chairs

Chairs can help or hinder the maintenance of a client's independence. Very few people have the same measurements in relation to thigh length or trunk depth but chairs are rarely designed to suit the individual. The vast majority of chairs are mass-produced so they are designed for the average user, and usually this is the average male. Ideally there should be space for gluteal muscles to bulge as they are compressed by the chair seat. We should be able to sit with our feet flat on the floor, without pressure under the lower third of the thigh and with our lumbar spine supported by the backrest.

If chairs are too low they will make it difficult or even impossible for the client to stand reasonably independently particularly if the hips are lower than their knees. When they are too high only the client's toes may be able to touch the floor, when the seat is too deep the client may be unable to relax against the backrest unless they are right back in the seat. In both of these instances the seat will exert pressure under the lower third of the thigh and back of the knee, where there is a large collection of blood vessels. The client will wriggle to relieve the pressure on these vessels. This wriggling to relieve the pressure is one of the causes of people sliding down their chairs. To relieve the pressure at the back of the knees or lower third of the thighs a low footstool or variable height footrest can be used. Be careful not to raise the feet too high or make the angle at the knees greater than 90 degrees (right angle).

When sitting the hips should be at least on the same level as the knees or preferably slightly above.

Chair raisers

These can be used to raise a chair height by 5–12.5 cm. There are two varieties. One type, suitable for chairs such as dining room chairs and stools, has sleeves which fit over the legs of the chair. The other is suitable for armchairs and has four sockets fitted to a frame. If using a hoist with this type of chair raiser take care that you ensure the hoist legs fit around the chair. It has been known for a hoist to become wedged under a chair fitted with a frame. **It is unsafe to use separate blocks or any other article to raise chairs or beds.**

Chairs that actively assist standing

These chairs are widely available. Some people who have arthritis or weak thigh muscles, but who can weight bear when standing, purchase their own. There is a wide variety of chairs where either the seat rises and tilts or the whole chair rises and tilts. Chairs where the whole chair moves are electrically operated using a hand-held control. A hazard notice has been issued for some electrically operated chairs because of a fatal injury to a child when a user operated the control to lower the chair and was unaware that the child was behind them.

These chairs should not be used for any person who has no sitting balance or head control.

Hoists

The use of a hoist (Fig. 7.4) should be planned into client care and not be an afterthought or due to an unexpected situation. There are many different makes and models of hoist available and they do not all have the same function. You need to be sure of the functions of the hoist supplied to your working area. Will it raise a client from a sitting to a standing position which requires the client to be able to hold on, weight bear on at least one leg and follow instructions? Or is it a sling-lifting hoist, which could be used to lift a fallen client from the floor? Some sling-lifting hoists can also be used to lift a client in a supine position, using either a frame or a split stretcher. All hoists have a weight limit and you need to know that limit. You need to practise with the hoist provided so that you are proficient in its use.

Hoists can be fixed, mobile, ceiling mounted or occasionally on a gantry or A-frame. They can be manually operated or powered, usually by battery.

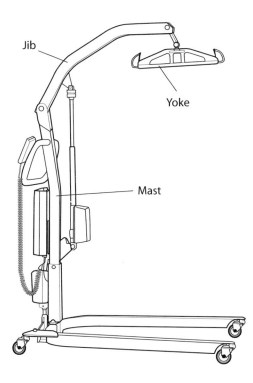

Fig. 7.4 A hoist.

Manually operated hoists raise the user either by the action of a hydraulic pump or by a winding handle. Both of these can strain the arms and shoulders of the operator as the weight of the client is being raised by the effort of the relatively weak muscle of arms and upper back. The power system of a powered hoist raises the weight of the client but both still have to be moved by the effort of the operator. Many of the newer hoists have been made lighter by the use of modern materials, but they still need weight to maintain their stability. It should be remembered that the operator is pushing the combined weight of the client and the hoist. They are therefore best used to transfer clients across a small distance such as bed to wheelchair rather than transport the client from the bed to another area.

Hoist slings

The sling should be suitable for the client. Most manufacturers will modify their own slings for clients who have specific difficulties. You need to estimate the most accurate weight for the client. A weight estimate of 140 kg for a client who weighed 102 kg resulted in the use of an extra-large sling which was potentially dangerous for client and staff. A client who is tall and slim may need a larger size of sling to manage extra trunk length safely. Some manufacturers recommend that if you need to raise a client from the floor you need a sling that is a size larger for the client than is normally used. Toileting slings sometimes need to be one size smaller than the general-purpose sling that the client would normally use. Always check with the client's care plan and the available literature for that particular hoist. You need to ensure that the sling being used for the client is compatible with the hoist. Many hoist manufacturers stipulate that only slings supplied by them and designed for their particular range of hoists should be used with their hoists.

To assist in infection control some hoist companies are supplying one-user only slings. These slings should remain with the client and should not be used for any one else or be washed. They should be replaced if soiled. **Remember: no sling should go from one person to another without first being washed in accordance with the manufacturer's instructions and infection control protocols.**

Principles of hoist use

Always push a hoist by its handle or mast and never push it by its jib as it may become unbalanced. The hoist must be suitable for the task, e.g. do not use a standing and raising hoist for someone who cannot weight bear or a 150 kg limit hoist for a client who weighs 180 kg. The majority of general-purpose slings are a modified C-shape and can be placed on the person in either a sitting or a lying position.

1. Ensure that the hoist will work with the chair or bed. The legs of the hoist should be able to fit under the bed and not collide with, or obstruct, the raising and lowering mechanism. When transferring into a chair the legs should spread sufficiently to allow the hoist to place the user at the back of the chair.
2. Place the sling on the client with the bed raised to the height most suitable for yourself and any colleague working with you.
3. Once the sling is on the client, ensure that the bed is at its lowest level before taking the client to or from the bed.
4. Raise the hoist just enough to remove the client from the bed or chair. It is frightening for the client to be more than a chair seat above the ground when a hoist is being manoeuvred.
5. When a hybrid hoist is provided, i.e. a different jib is used for a different task, ensure that the jib is secured in position.
6. When using a powered hoist ensure that the battery is re-charged well before it runs out. Don't leave it to someone else as someone else usually turns into no-one else.

Frames

Standing frames

These are designed to enable the person who has some strength in their thigh muscles to pull themselves up to a standing position. The usual design is to have a solid base plate on which the client places both feet plus a handle that the client can use to pull themselves upright. Some have a turning device which allows the base plate to rotate so that clients may, for example, stand on their own from a bed, be turned round by the care worker, then sit themselves down on a nearby

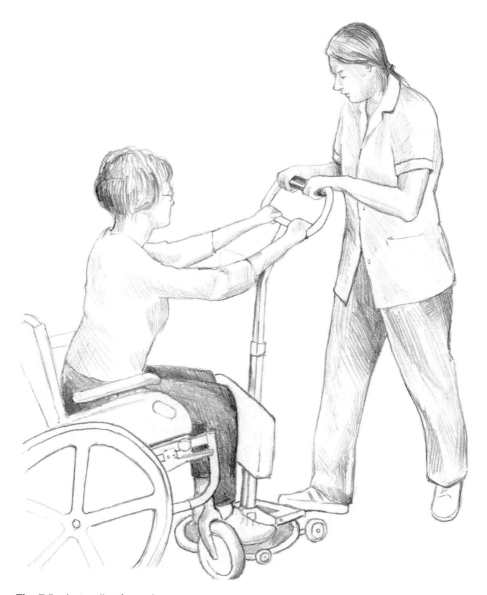

Fig. 7.5 A standing frame in use.

commode or wheelchair without the carer taking the weight when the client stands or supporting them as they sit. This allows the client to use the residual abilities they may have and helps to preserve some independence.

Walking frames

These are sometimes referred to as 'Zimmer' frames. Walking frames are intended to be picked up and moved forward, so are far lighter and not as stable as standing frames. As a result **they are not safe or suitable for clients to use to pull themselves from a sitting to a standing** position. They are intended to assist the person who needs assistance with balance or a little extra support when walking. The person using a walking frame should first stand, or be helped to stand, and then be handed the walking frame. Most walking frames have a maximum user weight of 125 kg (20 stone). Make sure the frame is the correct height for the client. There are also two-, three- and four-wheeled versions available. If a client needs to use an aid such as a frame, walking stick or crutches, ensure that the rubber ferrules on the bottom of the crutch, frame or stick still have their pattern on them and that they haven't worn smooth.

Trapezes (sometimes known as monkey poles)

These are a common sight in many hospital wards and there are models suitable for home use. Do not assume that everyone can use them to pull him- or herself up or move him- or herself backwards. They need strong arm, shoulder and abdominal muscles to be able to lift body weight, plus strong thigh muscles to push themselves backwards. As the muscles tend to weaken with age the elderly client is less likely to be able to use Trapezes. As the shoulder and arm muscles of females are considered to be 60% weaker than those of the equivalent male they are also less likely to be able to use them.

Sliding systems

Friction hinders movement so sliding systems aim to overcome friction by the use of low friction materials. They can be used to slide from one horizontal surface to another, e.g. bed to chair or trolley to bed or assist a client to move back up a bed. Some systems are multidirectional while others will slide in one direction only. There are three main categories of sliding systems: rigid boards, fabric-covered roller boards and fabric slides.

Boards and rollers

These come in assorted shapes and sizes. Small ones that may be straight or slightly curved are suitable for independent transfer of a client with sitting balance from one surface to another. Larger boards are suitable for the transfer of supine clients from one horizontal surface to another. The advantage of large, rigid boards is that they can bridge a slight gap of 75–150 mm (3–6 inches). The main disadvantages are that, if not inserted correctly, they can damage a client's tissue; they are somewhat unwieldy and the transfer may come to an abrupt stop once the bulk of the client's body is off the board and on the higher-friction material of a sheet covering the bed or trolley.

Fabric systems

These can also come in assorted sizes and styles. They can be single sheets, a continuous roll of single fabric, or quilted rolls like open-ended sleeping bags.

They can be used for a variety of tasks such as moving clients up and down the bed, turning and for re-positioning the client into the middle of the bed if they have just sat down on the bed. The full-length quilted slide can be used for turning clients on to their sides or for sideways horizontal transfers. Clients, particularly thin ones, tend to find these more comfortable than the rigid boards. They can be used when there is a small (no more than 75 mm) gap, but not if the gap is wider.

General principles

- Always have the surface the client is being transferred from slightly higher than the one that the client is rolling on to. You need to remember when transferring from a bed that the client's weight will depress the mattress quite considerably and the heavier the client the deeper the depression at the edge of the mattress when the client reaches that point. Allowance must be made for this when positioning the bed prior to the transfer otherwise the client may be bruised by the hard edge of the trolley and the resistance of the bed or trolley mattress may cause difficulties for the staff.
- Use body weight transfer when pushing or pulling. (See section on use of body weight.)
- Pushing should commence before pulling to avoid leaning across a bed or trolley in order to pull the client towards their destination.
- Do not use draw or single sheets when using large boards for a horizontal transfer. They are not made of low friction material, can be old, weakened by washing and bleaching agents in detergents and their tensile strength has not been tested. It is safer to use sliding sheets with lengthened handles.
- Do not use sheets – single sheets or draw sheets – with small transfer boards. They can be caught on chairs and wheelchairs, which may result in the client landing on the floor. If the client needs to have fabric underneath them a **small** handtowel folded to fit the board can be used, or some companies provide a special pad.
- Small transfer boards should not be used for sitting transfer for clients who have no sitting balance.
- Poles and canvas should never be used for a horizontal transfer.
- A manual lift, even using three, four or five people, should not be used for a horizontal transfer.

References

1. Department of Employment (1974) *Health and Safety at Work Act 1974*. HMSO, London.
2. Health and Safety Executive (1998) *Management of Health and Safety at Work: Approved Code of Practice 1992* and *1998*. HMSO, London.
3. Health and Safety Executive (1998) *Manual Handling Operations Regulations 1992* and *1998*. HMSO, London.

4. Health and Safety Executive (1998) *Manual Handling, Guidance on the Regulations MHOR 1992 and 1998*. HMSO, London.
5. Health Services Advisory Committee working group report (1992 and 1998) *The Manual Handling of Loads in the Health Services 1992 and 1998*. HMSO, London.
6. Health and Safety Executive (1998) *Provision and Use of Work Equipment Regulations 1992 and 1998*. HMSO, London.

Further reading

Back Care at Work. An Ergonomic Guide to Manual Handling. (1991) National Back Pain Association, Teddington. (This book is aimed at those who undertake risk assessments or are safety representatives as well as managers and supervisors.)

Handling People: Equipment, Advice, Information, 2nd edition (2001) Disabled Living Foundation, London. Website:www.dlf.org.uk

Kroemer, K.H.E. and Grandjean, E. (1997) *Fitting the Task to the Human. A Textbook of Occupational Ergonomics,* 5th edition. Taylor and Francis, USA (See Chapter 1.2 on static work and Chapters 7.1 and 7.2 on manual handling.)

Pheasant, S. (1991) *Ergonomics, Work and Health.* Palgrave Macmillan, UK. (See Chapter 15, p. 227 onwards: a discussion on lifting and handling.)

Oliver, J. and Middleditch, A. (1991) *Functional Anatomy of the Spine.* Butterworth Heinemann, Oxford. (A very good text if you want to know more about the way the spine functions. Can be 'dipped into'.)

Royal College of Nursing (2004) *RCN Guidance on Professional Matters for Health Care Assistants and Nurse Cadets.* Royal College of Nursing, London.

Safer Handling in the Community: Back Care. The National Back Pain Association, Teddington (A useful book for care workers assisting people in their own homes.)

The Handling of Patients: A Guide for Nurses, (Revised) 4th edition (1998) Back Care – National Back Pain Association (Teddington) in conjunction with the Royal College of Nursing, London. (A definitive guide for health professionals to cover risk assessment and ergonomics of handling patients.)

Chapter 8
Mobility and safer client handling

Fay Reid

This chapter follows on from the previous one, Chapter 7. The overview and keywords for Chapter 7 are relevant to both chapters. This Chapter expands on the issues and legislation discussed in Chapter 7 and their application to the practicalties of client care. It should be read after Chapter 7.

Assisting people to move

When you are moving a client *always* explain what you are going to do and seek the client's co-operation. You may find it helpful to ask the client to take a deep breath in when you say 'steady' and to breathe out when you say, 'stand' or whatever activity you are carrying out.

Before you attempt to move clients always check with the care plan, or whatever form of documentation there is for the client. Mobility and risk assessments should have been completed during the assessment of the client. This risk assessment is not the same as the assessment of the risk for the client of developing pressure sores. **The mobility risk assessment is an assessment of the risk of any injury to staff that might occur when staff have to help the client to move.**

The client's mobility assessment should tell you if:

- The client can weight bear through both, or only one, leg
- If they can only weight bear through one leg – which one?
- They have sitting and standing balance
- Their thigh muscles are sufficiently strong for them to be able to stand from sitting without anyone else taking their weight
- The client has a tendency to fall or any problem that might increase the risk of them falling
- They remember and can follow instructions
- They are **always** co-operative
- There is any tendency for them to be aggressive

The care plan should give you information on:

- What the client can manage without assistance, e.g. Mrs Brown can sit without support

- What assistance is needed, e.g. may need reminding of the moves needed to reach edge of bed. Bed should be slightly above her knee height to allow her to stand more easily
- What technique and/or equipment to use, e.g. can stand using a standing aid and walk using her own frame. Needs someone to walk behind her to give her confidence at this stage and ensure she is using frame correctly. Will need wheelchair to toilet especially in the evening
- How many carers may be needed, e.g. can manage with one carer

The care plan should also indicate if the client's abilities vary throughout the day. Some people with low blood pressure may have difficulty if they are taken to a standing position too quickly in the morning. Others are far more forgetful in the evening when tired, and tired limbs may also drag.

It is important that you know what and how much clients can do for themselves so that you can encourage them to do it. They have a right to independence, to continue to do for themselves those activities which they can manage. They should not be conditioned into dependence because it is quicker to do something for them rather than allowing them to do it for themselves.

Risk assessment

A risk assessment of the task you are undertaking should be available for you to read. The assessment of the level of risk of injury to staff should follow an objective analysis of the task being undertaken for the client. It is unrealistic to expect every single task for every individual client to be assessed so the commonest activities undertaken every day for the majority of clients will probably have had a generic assessment and that is then applied to the individual factors for each person in their environment. The individual capability of the worker may also influence the risk of injury. It is acknowledged that manual handling may affect a pregnant worker adversely and there will be a system to reduce that risk. It is generally accepted that the worker aged under 20 or over the age of 50 years is more vulnerable because of the immaturity of the musculo-skeletal system on the one hand and reducing muscle strength owing to the effect of ageing on the other.

Custom and practice

Beware of custom and practice. When someone says 'But we always do it like this here' and you have been taught that the method 'always' used has a high risk of injury for the staff, say politely that you have been told it is unsafe and do not do it. Remember that many people suffer pain and injury because they followed what is 'always' done. For example, a very common task care assistants are asked to do is to help someone to stand from chairs or beds. Although it has been known for at least 20 years that supporting a client's weight by their shoulder is painful for them and there is a risk of injury for both client and carer, it can still be seen in use in homes and hospitals. This method of moving someone up a bed or to and from a sitting position has a number of names: axillary, drag, through-arm, or under-arm lift. **All of them are unsafe**.

Analysis of under-arm techniques

All the techniques mentioned above involve putting the care worker's arm under the client's shoulder. In order to do this, when the client is seated, the worker has to stoop. When someone leans forward to put their arm under the client's axilla, the extensor muscles of the back are working to stop them falling. The muscles are not contracting and then relaxing; they are held still. This static work prevents the trunk from responding to the effect of gravity and muscles of the back, buttocks and legs are involved. If the care worker then puts an arm around the client's back a twist is added to the stoop. In addition the arms are having to be supported against the effect of gravity.

One of the muscles in the back is the latissimus dorsi. It is a broad, triangular-shaped muscle which is attached to the spinous processes, the bony bumps of the lower thoracic, lumbar and sacral vertebrae that you can feel in your back. This muscle is attached to the lower ribs as well as the iliac crest. Its main functions are to extend the upper arm forward and adduct (move it towards the centre of the body) posteriorly. The latissimus dorsi is therefore involved in dynamic and static work simultaneously. With such a loose, flexible joint the worker has to exert considerable upward force under the client's shoulder, which will simply move upwards. Only when the shoulder can move no more will the force start to take the client forwards and upwards.

For the client there are a number of possible results. Frequently, the client feels pain and will cry out, particularly if they are confused. If they feel they are being pulled forwards and may fall they will attempt to put a foot forward to stop this happening. Should the client have had a stroke with loss of power in one leg then the only leg that can be moved is the unaffected one. The upward force under the client's axilla encourages them to think that the care workers are capable of taking all their weight, so they will relax and tend to sag. Both of these situations will result in much, if not all, the weight of the client being suspended on the carer's arms.

With a through-arm hold the care worker's hand is seldom able to hold the upper aspect of the forearm securely with a relaxed palm. It has been known for this hold to fracture a bone in the lower arm.

Standing a client when using any of these methods does not follow, or help to reinforce, the memory of the normal patterns of standing. Nor does it allow people to use or retain the strength remaining in their thigh muscles. Physiotherapists use a graded test for power in the thigh muscles and in order to be able to stand from sitting the client's muscles should reach at least grade 4. This means that the client's thigh muscles must have sufficient power to move the limb against gravity and some resistance. This is usually tested by asking the client to raise the leg while sitting while the physiotherapist applies resistance with the pressure of a hand on the knee. If the client cannot raise the leg while a hand is pressing on the knee then the thigh muscle has insufficient power to lift the trunk upwards against the effect of gravity. They will not be able to stand from the sitting position without the care worker taking some or all of their weight. Therefore, this situation gives rise to a foreseeable risk of injury to the care worker, and another means of transfer to a chair, such as a sliding board, providing the client can sit unsupported, should be used.

Holding a client

Use a wide, open relaxed palm to hold the client if you are guiding or assisting them to move. A tense hand may convey nervousness and anxiety to the client. In addition, some clients, particularly those taking aspirin or warfarin, may have finger mark bruising where they have been held tightly. If you have to support a client's limb, remember to hold the arm or leg above and below a joint. To pick arms and legs up and hold them in the air at just one point is painful for the client and could be harmful for you. Legs can be heavy: 15.7% of the body weight. This is approximately 12.31 kg (2 stone approx.) for the average male and it is not always possible to get close to lift them. If it is possible, stand level with the client's knee with bent knees, spine in alignment and keeping the spinal curves. Have as long a walking stride stance as the bed or trolley will allow. Slide one hand above the joint and the other below it. Allowing your head to lead the movement, straighten your knees. It is sometimes helpful to rest the client's foot or hand on your shoulder but ensure that you protect your clothing from potential contamination.

Sitting a client up

If the task of sitting someone up is analysed, the worker is supporting the weight of the client from hip joints upwards against the effect of gravity and raising them to sitting height. The weight of the average British woman aged between 18 and 65 years is 62.5 kg. The average man in the same age range weighs 74.5 kg. With trunk, head and arms accounting for 63% of the client's weight, the weight range for the average man and woman being supported is 41.6–49.6 kg. A box of five reams of paper weighs 12 kg and a standard bag of cement weighs 25 kg. While engaged in this task the worker is standing at the side of a 900-mm (3 feet) wide bed and will have to stoop and, in all probability, twist when supporting a client who is lying down.

Many clients find it difficult to sit up from a semi-supine position. This may be due to recent surgery, abdominal girth, poor balance or general muscle weakness and frailty. It can be extremely painful following surgery to be pulled up into a sitting position. Where possible, prior to surgery, ensure that the client knows how to sit up by bending knees, rolling to the side and pushing up with the hands. This may be more difficult if the client has a drainage tube in the wound area and infusions in their arms. However, it is far less painful for the client than being pulled upwards, in what is effectively a straight leg sit up, which puts tension on the abdominal muscles.

If clients cannot sit up by themselves then they should preferably be in an electrically operated bed whose backrest can be raised and the mattress platform positioned to support and maintain the client's position. However, a number of homes and hospitals do not have powered beds so there may be no option but to re-position the client using a manual technique. In this situation take either a handling sling, a slide sheet where the tensile strength has been identified, or the client's own towel folded lengthways into three and position it carefully behind the client's shoulders. This gives greater leverage and allows the client to be pulled upwards into a sitting position. Use a walking stride posture and transfer body weight from front to back foot. Do not attempt this on your own, as you will be raising and supporting a weight far in excess of the Health and Safety Executive's guidance, with both a twisted posture and an extended arm. As a last resort, if handling sling, sliding sheet or towel are not available then the bottom sheet can be used. If the client does not have sitting balance then a second person should support the client while pillows are re-arranged.

Some clients can use a rope ladder attached to the foot of the bed to pull themselves up to a sitting position. However, this may leave the client sitting a long way from the back-rest and pillows and then you are faced with the task of moving him or her back up the bed towards the backrest. A portable back-rest is useful in this situation. **No client should be manually lifted up the bed as this activity involves a high risk of injury to staff.**

Moving a client up the bed

How often have you been asked to help 'move a client up a bed'? This phrase is shorthand for 'We need to lift the client at least 15 cm to clear the bed. Carry them horizontally the required distance, lower them back to the mattress, while we are at arms length away from them.'

Activity 8.1

Moving back up a bed seems such a simple activity but let us analyse the movement involved for someone who is fit and mobile and then apply it to a frail, sick person. Sit on the floor, put your hands by your side and try to lift your trunk off the floor using only your arms to power the lift and support yourself. Now move yourself backwards without using your legs. Try the same activity sitting on a bed and you may find that you cannot clear the mattress because your weight has compressed the mattress and you are sitting in a slight dip. In addition, your hands sink into the mattress as well. When you try to move backwards you may not be able to because your arms are not long enough to overcome the extra distance you have to lift yourself. You may also be encountering some resistance from the mattress.

The safest way of managing the situation, particularly for heavy or very dependent clients would be to nurse them in an electrically operated profiling bed. On an ordinary King's Fund bed a one-way glide may reduce the frequency of the slide towards the bottom of the bed. Some clients may be able to use hand blocks, if they are available. The use of a sliding system may allow clients to slide themselves backwards. The client needs to be told to place their hands behind them, but not touching the slide. They are asked to place their feet flat on the mattress with knees bent. If the client has insufficient control over the lower limbs then the carer can help by blocking the feet to prevent them from sliding forwards and asking the client to push backwards. This process may be needed several times to re-position the client against the back-rest and pillows.

Turning a client in bed

There are occasions when a client will need to be turned in bed to allow access to their back or change the bottom sheet on the bed. **Never roll a client away from you unless there is a second person on the other side of the bed or side rails are in use and you have checked that they are safe and secure**. When the client is lying on their back in the bed there is approximately 237 mm (9 inches) on either side of the trunk. When turned onto a side from that position the depth of the abdomen will occupy most of the space so that they are effectively balanced at the edge of the bed. The bulk of the body weight is in front of the spine so there will be a tendency for gravity to pull them forward and therefore off the edge of the bed. This is a very frightening position to be in. In addition, they are lying on a very bony profile which is uncomfortable so they are likely to wriggle.

When supporting a client lying on a surface which is approximately 900 mm (3 feet) above the ground the care worker will have to lean forward in order to be able to place their arms down the back of the client. When doing this, the care workers are supporting approximately half their own body weight against the effect of gravity. At the same time the arms are raised to approximately shoulder level in order to place them down the back of the client. The latissimus dorsi muscle, which is involved in supporting the trunk against the effect of gravity is also involved in extending the arms and maintaining them in that position. The effect of holding this posture even for short periods of time may put a considerable strain on the muscles of the arms, back, neck and shoulders. Muscles whose normal activity is to contract and lengthen in order to move joints and limbs are held in a fixed state. This static muscle work, described in Chapter 7, is extremely fatiguing and can result in pain and eventual injury. The lower the bed the greater the risk to the care worker, particularly those who may be above average height. If the procedure being undertaken requires this position to be held for longer than a few minutes then staff should change roles to allow the muscles of the back and arms to rest and so reduce the risk.

Assisting a client to stand

When standing from a sitting position, thigh muscles have to be sufficiently strong to raise approximately two thirds of their total body weight. It is commonly accepted that human beings reach their maximum strength between 25 and 35 years. It is also widely recognised that women have about two-thirds the amount of muscle strength that men have and that muscles lose their strength as human beings age. Between the ages of 50 and 69 years people may only retain three-quarters of their former muscle strength; 75% of 65-year-old women cannot stand from a seated position without using their arms to push themselves up to a standing position.

When you know from the care plan or the assessment that the client can weight bear when standing, balance and walk safely, either on their own or with the aid of a walking stick or frame, ask yourself the question: 'Is the chair they are sitting in enabling or hindering them to stand?' Many elderly people can only stand from a sitting position by using the arms of their chairs. If you are holding them in such a way that they cannot use their arms then you will be taking some, or all, of their weight. The height of the seat is very important. If the chair is so low that the client's arms are fully extended before their thigh muscles can push them any higher or their knees and hips are flexed so that the hips are lower than knees, then standing independently is not possible without the care worker taking some or all of the weight.

When standing a client never allow them to clasp you behind the neck. Some clients who have had a stroke can go into backward extension; others with a very low blood pressure may fall. If this happens when they are holding on to you around the neck then their weight is going to be suspended on your cervical spine. Encourage the client to wriggle to the front of the chair. Ensure that both feet are flat on the floor, about hip distance apart. One foot should be forward with a right angle bend at the knee and the back foot will be against the edge of the chair with the knee bent at less than a right angle. The client leans forward from the hip so that the nose is above the toes and the head leads the standing movement. If the client's knees and hips are still bent by the time the arms have straightened and the person is unwilling or unable to let go of the chair's arms to stand, then you should ask for the client to be re-assessed. The client may find it easier to use a standing frame.

Walking a client

Stand on the weaker side of the client using a palm-to-palm hold. If you are on the client's left you will be holding his or her left hand with your left hand. This allows the hand that is nearest to the client to give support around the waist. You will need to walk very close to and slightly behind the client. In this position you will be in control of the situation and will able to take appropriate action should the client feel faint or fall. **Never attempt to catch or hold up a client who is falling**.

Technique for controlling a fall

The human body responds to the effect of gravity exactly like any other body if, for any reason, it ceases to be able to maintain an upright posture. The human body will fall at the rate of 9.8 metres (32.8 feet) per second. In areas where there are sick, frail or elderly people it is essential that there is a system for managing the falling or fallen person.

The aim of controlling the fall is to prevent or reduce the risk of injury to the client and the care worker. Most people falling forward, who are unconscious, or not quick enough to put their hands forward to help break their fall, tend to get head, facial and shoulder injuries. It should also help to prevent you from acquiring a very painful injury should you stoop and attempt to lower them to the floor. The technique allows the client to slide down your body so that their head does not strike the floor. This is a very skilled and complex manoeuvre and should only be demonstrated and taught by experienced practitioners in a safe environment, i.e. with a floor covered in thick exercise or crash mats.

The technique of allowing clients to slide to the floor is against the instincts of most care workers who try to prevent clients from injuring themselves. Should you feel the client sag and they do not respond to a command such as 'Keep standing', let go of their hand, slide your hands upwards to their axillae, and move behind them placing one leg forward with a bent knee. Should they continue to sag, lower your hands until your body is like a slide and allow them to slide down it to the floor. This at least prevents the client from hitting the floor face down and should prevent you from stooping and supporting their weight. This technique can only succeed when the care worker is standing so close that they are in direct physical contact with the client and their hand and arm are not trapped between the client's trunk and arm. It should only be practised with expert supervision and in a safe, protected environment.

Managing a client who has fallen

It is not uncommon for the elderly to fall. It is one of the commonest reasons for admission of the elderly to an accident and emergency unit. The causes are many and varied. They range from transient ischaemic and drop attacks; weakness of one or both legs; problems with special senses such as poor vision or vertigo; low blood pressure caused by dehydration or occasionally drugs such as beta-blockers, used to treat hypertension; and poor righting reflexes. These are just a few causes and they all increase the risk of the client falling. Any client's risk of falling should be recorded in the mobility assessment and known to all.

There are only three courses of action that can be taken for the person who has fallen to the floor, as **no client should ever be manually lifted from the floor**. Very few able people who fall rush to get up themselves up from the floor. It is usually others who hurry to pull them up. The person who has fallen generally likes to get his or her breath back, checks that no great damage has been done and tries to regain some sort of composure before they stand themselves up.

Many people like to get their breath back before making the effort to get up as hitting the ground frequently winds them. Make them as comfortable as possible, ensure they have suffered no injury and when they are ready:

- Encourage them to get themselves up if they can follow instructions or demonstration, or
- Use a lifting cushion to take the person to chair or bed height, or
- Use a hoist

To get themselves off the floor someone who is uninjured should bend their knees, roll to their side and then on to their hands and knees. A chair is very helpful for the person trying to stand as the seat can be used to help push up to a standing, or sitting, position. The person who lives alone and is prone to fall should be taught how to get up from the floor. The instruction should include giving written information with clear diagrams to act as a reminder.

Bathing

It is far easier to get into a bath than to get out of one. In order to get out of the bath strength in thigh muscles, balance and four fully functioning limbs are needed. **No person should be routinely manually lifted out of a bath**. There is a variety of means for getting into and out of baths. These range from hoists to bath seats and raising aids. The client should have been assessed to identify the most suitable type of assistance.

Activity 8.2

Get into a dry bath and then get out of it thinking what your arms and legs are doing in order to get you into a standing position so you can step out. Then sit down again and try to get out while your right hand is on your left shoulder or around your waist. Think what would happen if one of your knees would not bend. You have also got to be able to lift legs high enough to allow feet to go over the side of the bath (which is approximately 400 mm [16 inches])

Bath seats are sometimes given to enable people to use a bath who may not have the ability to get out of a bath easily. The minimum height of most of these seats is 152 mm (6 inches) and the thigh thickness of an 'elderly person' when seated is about 145 mm (5.5 inches). The water level would need to be almost level with the overflow pipe to cover the client's thighs. If they move off the bath seat to get their trunk into the warm water they must have sufficient strength in their arms and shoulders to be able to raise themselves back onto the bath seat. If the client cannot raise their buttocks from the seat of a chair when pushing up with hands on the seat it is unlikely that they will be able to lift themselves onto a bath seat from the bath. If they have to sit and balance on a bath board or the edge of the bath, sitting balance is needed, otherwise they may fall.

If there is a shower attachment available the bath seat does make it easy to shower in the bath. However, many people find a shower colder and less comforting than a bath.

Toileting

One of the major problems when toileting clients is the lack of space in most toilet cubicles or bathrooms. This may be particularly true in the residential home or domestic environment. An independent wheelchair user should be able to access the WC pan from either side of the WC as not everyone transfers off and onto their wheelchairs from the same side. Toilets for dependent wheelchair users should have sufficient space, at least 900 mm (3 feet) on either side of the WC pan to enable care workers to assist the wheelchair user without the need to work in an awkward posture. Two people who are trying to assist a third need enough space to let everyone involved move freely without having to bend or twist. Two or three people in a toilet area designed for an independent individual is a common cause of injury to staff.

There are many aids to assist toileting including hand rails, both vertical and horizontal, raised toilet seats, toileting hoists and toileting slings for use with sling lifting hoists. The use of mobile hoists in a toilet or bathroom will require sufficient space and suitable floor covering for the hoist to be manoeuvred easily with the client in it.

Team handling

Do not be tempted to use people to move the client manually and without equipment if you cannot find the equipment specified in the care plan. **Do not assume that more equals safe**. Two people do not have the same capability as the total of two individuals' capability. A team need more space and lack of sufficient space in which to move will also increase the risk of injury for everyone involved in the activity. The team must also move in unison to avoid the hazard of an unsynchronised lift. We do not naturally move in unison, nor have we been drilled to do so as chorus lines or squads of guardsmen are.

Where two people are needed to assist a client do not assume because you have worked with someone previously that you both will automatically move in unison and there is no need to give a clear command. The client is also part of the team so explain to them what you are intending to do and continue to tell the client what you are going to do at every stage of the movement. Identify a leader, ensure everyone is ready and all commands should be given very clearly. 'Ready, steady, . . .' then whatever activity is going to follow such as 'slide' or 'stand'. This indicates to client and colleague exactly what you intend to do and is much clearer to everyone. Many nurses have been injured as a result of unsynchronised movements.

Chapters 7 and 8 on mobility have been included to enable you to follow safe principles when assisting other people to undertake their activities of daily living. All the information is based on recognised and available texts. The chapters indicated in the texts in the section further reading support and add to the information contained in this chapter. They provide essential information to develop your knowledge and skills.

Further reading

Department of Employment (1974) *Health and Safety at Work Act 1974.* HMSO, London.

Handling People, Equipment, Advice, Information, 2nd edition (2001) Disabled Living Foundation, London.

Health and Safety Executive (1998) *Management of Health and Safety at Work: Approved Code of Practice 1992* and *1998.* HMSO, London.

Health and Safety Executive (1998) *Manual Handling Operations Regulations 1992* and *1998.* HMSO, London.

Health and Safety Executive (1998) *Manual Handling, Guidance on the Regulations MHOR 1992* and *1998.* HMSO, London.

Health and Safety Executive (1998) *Provision and Use of Work Equipment Regulations 1992* and *1998.* HMSO, London

Health Services Advisory Committee working group report. (1992 and 1998) *The Manual Handling of Loads in the Health Services, 1992* and *1998.* HMSO, London.

Kroemer, K.H.E. and Grandjean, E. (1997) *Fitting the Task to the Human. A Textbook of Occupational Ergonomics*, 5th edition. Taylor and Francis, USA. (See chapter 1.2 on static work and Chapters 7.1 and 7.2 on manual handling.)

Oliver, J. (1998) *Back in Line.* Butterworth Heinemann, Oxford.

Pheasant, S. (1991) *Ergonomics, Work and Health.* Palgrave Macmillan, UK pp. 32, 33 and 37 on static and dynamic work and p. 43 on strength.

Royal College of Nursing (2004) *RCN Guidance on Professional Matters for Health Care Assistants and Nurse Cadets.* Royal College of Nursing, London.

The Handling of Patients: a Guide for Nurses (Revised) 4th edition (1997) Back Care – National Back Pain Association (Teddington) in conjunction with the Royal College of Nursing, London.

Chapter 9
Control of infection

Heather Rowe

Overview

Definition: infection is the invasion of the body by disease-causing organisms (germs). In our daily lives we pay little attention to the possibility of contracting a serious infection. There is almost an expectation that one may catch a cold in the winter season, and while inconvenient and uncomfortable for us, nonetheless it does not pose a serious threat to life.

Man has developed a phenomenal ability to interact with other humans, animals and the environment to enable us to enjoy a healthy existence. However, this is a fine balance that, if breached, may result in disease and/or infection.

Organisms that cause disease in man are called pathogens. The essential element of this chapter is to help you safeguard your health when caring for clients with infections. This knowledge is essential for you to implement safe care for a client, without adding the risk of them acquiring a hospital-borne infection.

Key words: Invasive procedure; micro-organisms; virus; bacteria; parasite; cross-infection; commensals; disinfectants; isolation; aseptic; clean; iatrogenic; pathogens; pathogenic; endogenous; exogenous; sterile; defence mechanisms; natural immunity; passive immunity

What causes infection?

Small living organisms, which can only be seen with a microscope – hence the word micro-organism – predominantly cause infection. Organisms can be further categorised along the lines of a family tree (Fig. 9.1). There are numerous names given to the organisms, according to their shape, size and behaviour. Staphylococci live on the human skin in harmony with the individual, doing no harm while they remain in that habitat. Only about 90% of organisms are potentially harmful to humans.

How do individuals keep infection-free?

The immune system is the mechanism by which humans resist infection. Some individuals, especially those already in poor health, are considered more

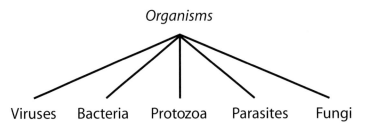

Fig. 9.1 Classification of micro-organisms.

susceptible to infection. Humans have a complex immune system that under most circumstances protects them against infection. Part of the immune system is a collection of specialised cells which are transported in the bloodstream and the lymphatic vessels to all parts of the body. The cells involved in this process are predominantly the white blood cells.

The body uses physiological processes to constantly monitor for infection. If infection is detected the body activates the immune system to combat the invasion of pathogens. In most instances the individual will be able to recover after a short illness. However, some individuals suffer considerably and many even die from hospital-acquired infections (HAI), that is to say the client develops an infection while being cared for which may arise from other patients or from the staff.

Defence mechanisms

- Juices in our digestive tract are designed to eliminate many of the harmful organisms which we ingest. The composition of juices alters along the digestive tract to ensure potentially harmful organisms are destroyed. For example, hydrochloric acid is produced in the stomach and most organisms are destroyed by acid.
- Tears constantly bathe the surface of our eyes to flush away organism-laden dust particles.
- Intact skin is a huge body defence against invasion by organisms. Keeping the skin in a healthy condition and free from cuts and abrasions is an important aspect of prevention of infection. Patients who develop decubitus ulcers (pressure sores) in fact have the wound infected by organisms, thus making the healing process considerably more difficult.

Immunity

Once the body has been exposed to a harmful (pathogenic) organism it usually produces an antibody cell to oppose and overcome that specific organism. If the person is exposed at a later time to the same organism, the antibody cell will remember and immediately multiply to combat this fresh invasion. It is only pathogenic organisms which are a potential danger to humans; that is to say those organisms which are capable of causing disease. The human body has many organisms that aid body functions while they are restricted in a specific area. For example, vitamin K production in the intestines is aided by bacterial activity. Such organisms are known as commensals or normal flora. Should the organisms colonise in another area of the body they are capable of causing an infection. Colonisation means the organisms multiply and flourish. For example, *Escherichia coli*, a commensal organism normally found in the bowel, may cause infection if it is transmitted to the urethra and ascends to the bladder.

Susceptibility of an individual to infection depends on the virulence of the organism, the number of organisms and the state of the individual's immune system.

Sources of pathogenic transmission

- Humans
- Insects
- Animals
- Inanimate objects

Humans

As previously discussed, numerous organisms are commensals and may be passed to another individual by direct or indirect contact. If an individual, be they nurse or client, has an infection, they may infect another individual by cross-infection, whether in the incubation phase, acute phase or convalescent period of the infection. Some individuals are carriers of particular organisms that do not cause infection in the carrier but harm others. For example a carrier of *Staphylococcus aureus* in their nose will not necessarily show signs of infection. However, the carrier is potentially harmful if caring for vulnerable patients. It is sometimes necessary for staff who work with such clients to have regular nasal swab tests to check they are free from infection.

Animals

Animals may cause infection in several ways. The commonest mode is when animals are consumed as food. Poultry is notorious for carrying the organism salmonella, which may cause food poisoning in humans.

Insects

A mosquito bite can cause malaria in some parts of the world.

Inanimate objects

Soil, water and air are all capable of supporting organisms. The tetanus organism inhabits the soil. *Vibrio cholerae*, which causes cholera, inhabits some water supplies. *Legionella pneumophila*, the cause of legionnaires' disease, can inhabit water- and air-cooling systems in buildings.

Modes of pathogenic transmission

There are two modes of transmission: direct and indirect.

Direct transmission

Contact between humans

This is an area where the carer needs to ensure that their own hygiene and habits are scrupulous, so as not to convey either their own organisms, or those of other clients, to another individual.

Inadequate handwashing between each client contact can lead to the spread of infection. For example, hands may become contaminated when emptying a urinary catheter bag; therefore, it is essential to wash one's hands after each client contact. Even though one wears gloves when dealing with patients' body fluids, it is still essential to wash your hands after any such procedure. It may be that hand rub solutions are available as an alternative to handwashing. The key point is that one's hands should be thoroughly cleaned after each patient episode. It is estimated that there are around 100000 instances of HAI each year which represents 1 in 11 patients at any one time[1]. This represents a huge amount of suffering for the patient as well as a considerable cost to the NHS. As part of the strategy to reduce this incidence effective handwashing is essential.

Transmission by inoculation

This is a risk in an accidental sharps injury. It is a particular risk when the damaging object, such as a needle or scalpel blade, is contaminated with blood or body fluids. This is one way of contracting hepatitis B. Prevention is the best practice, so always work to the current policy and procedures for the disposal of sharps.

Sexual contact

This is yet another mode of direct spread. As it is not an important aspect in the nursing of clients, it will not be dealt with any further here.

Indirect transmission

There are numerous modes of indirect spread and each one will be dealt with separately.

Droplet spread

This may occur when speaking, coughing or sneezing. Small water particles are formed and then sprayed into the atmosphere during these activities. These droplets, as they are called, may carry pathogenic or commensal organisms, which are inhaled by another individual. For example, the common cold is usually spread by droplet infection. A wound can be infected from a carer's commensal organisms that inhabit their nose and throat. Therefore, it is desirable to limit conversation during a wound dressing procedure.

Vectors

This term refers to carriers such as flies and cockroaches.

Fomites

This mode of infection is via inanimate objects. These are so numerous that it is important for the carer to understand the mode of transmission, rather than the objects involved. Examples include:

- Carers' uniforms
- Bedpans
- Eating utensils
- Toiletries
- Bedclothes
- All manner of equipment that may be used in the client's care

This is an area for significant concern as many of the procedures carried out in the work area are designed to prevent this mode of infection. For example, wearing a single use, disposable apron for stripping the linen off a used bed to prevent contamination of clothing which may come in contact with a client later on.

Activity 9.1

Consider one client you have cared for and list the inanimate objects that could cause the spread of infection.

Your list may include the following:

- Bedclothes
- Polythene washing bowl
- Bed cradle
- Pillows
- Towel
- Patient's lifting hoist

Airborne spread

The air suspends many organisms, thus facilitating the inhalation of organisms when we breathe. Therefore, one endeavours to reduce air currents in the work area to a minimum. It is essential to have fresh air, but not a draught. For example, fold the bed linen when stripping a used bed, as shaking and pulling create an air current and increase the circulation of organisms and dust.

Vulnerability to infection

Activity 9.2

Before reading further, spend a few minutes considering the factors you can iden-tify which predispose people to infection.
 Now read on and see how many you were able to identify.

Factors which increase the risk of infection are shown in Fig. 9.2.

Age

At either end of the continuum one is less able to resist infection. The very young have an immature immune system, while in older people the immune system

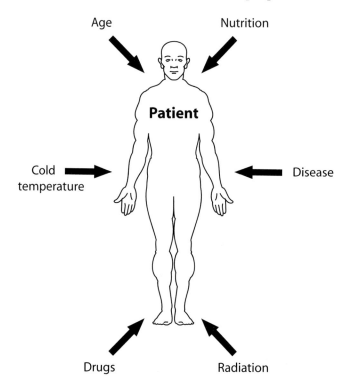

Fig. 9.2   Factors which increase the risk of infection.

tends to no longer respond rapidly to infection. For example, food poisoning may give an otherwise healthy person severe diarrhoea and vomiting, but could well prove fatal for an older person or the young.

Nutrition

Malnutrition predisposes individuals to infection, as they are unable to produce antibodies effectively. This is especially true when there is a lack of protein in the diet.

Low temperature

Exposure to temperatures which reduce the core body temperature to below normal is thought to suppress antibody production. For example, the exposure of wounds and the use of solutions reduce the healing capacity for several hours.

Disease

Individuals who are already ill may have an inefficient immune system, increasing their susceptibility to infection. This applies especially to individuals suffering from diseases such as diabetes mellitus, cancer or acquired immune deficiency syndrome (AIDS).

Drugs

Some drugs, especially the corticosteroids (e.g. prednisolone), while essential for controlling some diseases nonetheless suppress antibody production. For example, clients receiving chemotherapy drugs for the treatment of cancer are more susceptible to infection because of their drug regimen.

Radiation

Exposure to therapeutic doses of radiation reduces the body's ability to produce antibodies and white blood cells.

Care of the client with an infection

One aim is to increase the client's resistance to the infection. They are likely to need a nutritious diet, high in calories and protein. The client frequently does not feel like eating and drinking, so the carer needs to be imaginative in finding tempting morsels. Often special high-calorie and protein drinks are ideal; perhaps these could be made into ice blocks for the patient to suck, or if the taste is unpalatable provide a drinking straw.

Because the client usually has a raised body temperature they require extra fluid to replace that lost by sweating. This is likely to be about 2500–3000 ml per day. The carer can, by encouragement, do a great deal to ensure the client consumes this large volume of fluid. Help the client to rest as much as possible by promoting an environment conducive to sleep. Comfort is important so change damp bed linen as necessary. Cotton night attire is best as it causes the least sweating. The client may feel alternately hot and cold, as body temperature fluctuates. A fan will help during the hot flush period and blankets when the patient feels cold. It is important to prevent shivering as this consumes a lot of energy. Figure 9.3 illustrates factors which help fight infection.

Inflammation

This is the body's response to infection and may be observed by the carer. If any of the symptoms shown in Fig. 9.4 are observed, or mentioned by the client, it is important to inform the registered practitioner. These signs and symptoms are the result of the immune response and evidence that the body is responding to the pathogens and trying to combat the infection and destroy the harmful organisms.

Management of the client with an infection

The aim of the care is not only to allow the client to recover, **but also to prevent the spread of the infection to others: yourself, other staff or other clients**. It is also important that the infected client is not exposed to another infection caused through inadequate preventive care. This latter type of infection is referred to as cross-infection, and hospitalised patients are especially vulnerable to contracting such infections (HAI). However, vigilance with regard to personal hygiene and the correct carrying out of procedures can reduce the risks considerably.

One such HAI is caused by methicillin-resistant *Staphylococcus aureus* (MRSA). This micro-organism is commonly found on the skin, especially in the axilla and perineum area as well as the nose. The carrier comes to no harm from the micro-organism; however, if it is transferred to a vulnerable patient by direct contact with the skin or contaminated equipment or environment, their illness may become life-threatening. Resistance relates to the fact that antibiotics are no longer effective in eradicating the micro-organism.

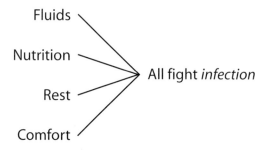

Fig. 9.3 Factors which help in the fight against infection.

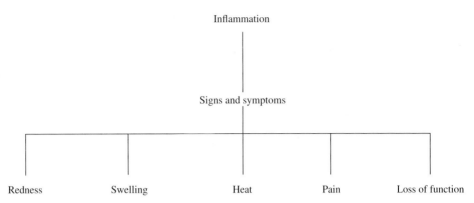

Fig. 9.4 Signs and symptoms of inflammation.

Source isolation nursing

If the client already has an infection that is virulent, that is to say the pathogen is extremely likely to cause infection in another client, then they may be isolated in the hope of preventing such spread to other patients and staff. For example, some clients who have a severe wound infection or tuberculosis will be isolated. The ward manager will ascertain who is safe to care for this client. In general, if you have been immunised for tuberculosis then you can safely care for the client.

Specific procedures will be followed for clients in isolation regarding the disposal of waste materials and the movement of personnel and equipment within the nursing area. Refer to the local policy for specific details to ensure safe practice. These procedures will be supported by your local infection control nurse. If in any doubt always consult a specialist nurse.

Protective isolation

Other clients in isolation are those who must be protected from receiving an infection from others or the environment. For example, this is anyone receiving special drug therapy that greatly reduces their ability to produce antibodies and other immune defence mechanisms. These clients are susceptible to contracting infection from anybody or anything with which they come into contact. They are nursed in rooms where the ventilation and temperature are ideally controlled.

All inanimate objects entering the area will be sterile. A sterile object is one that is free from all organisms. There are various ways to make objects sterile, usually involving heat, disinfectants or radiation treatment. Personnel will usually wear protective sterile clothing, and possibly masks, to prevent the client receiving any of their airborne or droplet organisms.

Common risk factors for clients in hospital

- Shared facilities and equipment
- Contact with hospital staff

- Invasive procedures, e.g. surgery/endoscopy
- Mass-produced food
- High psychological stress factors
- Intravenous infusion
- Failure to adhere to vigilant handwashing technique

Prevention of cross-infection

- Individualised client care
- Hospital organisational policies and approaches designed to reduce infection
- Staff and client education

Individualised client care

Individualised care is acheived by assessing each individual, recording the assessment and planning the care accordingly. The care plan should always be consulted before care is given and the subsequent outcome of the care should be recorded. This enables efficient monitoring and evaluation of the client's condition.

Likewise, if a system of client allocation is practised it helps to reduce the number of personnel who come into contact with the client, thus reducing the client's risk of contracting an infection.

Hospital/trust organisational policies and procedures

The local policies and procedures should be current and available as guides for staff practices.

Activity 9.3

Identify the following in your work area: infection control policy, procedure manual.

Staff and client education

Clients may contract an infection from either themselves, termed endogenous, or from other sources, termed exogenous.

Endogenous infections frequently arise because the client is unaware of the hazards they expose themselves to. The client's commensal organisms can be spread to cause infection. For example, *Escherichia coli* from the perineum may cause a urinary tract infection in the patient who has not been taught the importance of perineal toilet following a bowel motion. The perineum is the area between the anus and the urethra (the opening to the bladder). This is especially important for the female client, as their urethra is short and, therefore, in close proximity to the anus. It is important to teach patients to clean their perineal area from front to back, thus preventing contamination from the anus.

Clients whose hands are contaminated with organisms may peel the corner of their wound dressing to have a look and in the process contaminate their wound. Teaching clients good hygiene habits and helping them to carry them out is part of the carer's role.

Activity 9.4

Record the facilities available for your clients to wash their hands following toileting.

For mobile clients the facilities for handwashing should include:

- Hot running water
- Individually dispensed soap solution
- Hand drying facilities with disposable towel and flip lid bin

For bed-bound clients these should include:

- Client's own soap
- Clean bowl of water
- Disposable flannel
- Hand towel
- Disposable handwipes

Exogenous infections are those acquired from others and/or the environment. The single most important preventive measure is scrupulous handwashing and drying technique by all personnel. Refer to your local policy and evidence from the literature.

General principles of handwashing

Taps can be heavily contaminated with organisms. It is important to use elbow taps correctly when they are available, that is, turn the taps on and off using your elbows (Fig. 9.5), or disposable paper towel, as this reduces the level of contamination on the taps and prevents re-contamination of your freshly washed hands. The general technique for handwashing is:

1. Remove wristwatch and jewellery.
2. Use hot running water to dampen your hands.
3. Use the correct amount of individually dispensed soap solution.
4. Thoroughly wash all areas of your hands, including under a wedding ring.
5. Rinse off soap.
6. Dry your hands thoroughly with disposable towels.

Handwashing before and after client contact is the single most important practice in the prevention of cross-infection. Clients' personal effects should not be

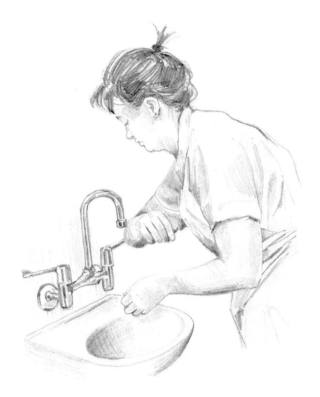

Fig. 9.5   Good handwashing technique.

loaned to other patients. Facecloths and soaps should be allowed to dry between usage, as this helps to reduce the environmental conditions which most organisms need for growth, that is, dampness and darkness.

Single-use items

Single-use, disposable items should be used whenever possible. However, this may be cost prohibitive or not accepted current practice. It is the carer's responsibility to make items available for the client and to ensure they are aware of safe usage and disposal.

Activity 9.5

In your work area, what facilities are available for clients to use headphone sets to listen to the radio? Are the earpieces disposable and changed, or cleaned if not disposable, between each client use?

Activity 9.6

Is there a sphygmomanometer used in your clinical area? If so how is the cleanliness of the arm cuff dealt with in terms of prevention of infection?

If material is not disposable but needs to be shared, then it is essential for the carer to understand the proper care for the equipment to prevent cross-infection. On the whole, the use of general purpose detergent and hot water for washing, followed by thorough drying, is appropriate for cleaning beds, bed cradles, etc., to control infection. Refer to your own organisational infection control policy.

Environment

All carers have a responsibility to ensure that the environment within which they work is as clean as possible, to prevent the growth of organisms. Damp, dark, unclean areas support colonisation; Florence Nightingale identified the importance of eradicating such conditions.

Pathogens may grow wherever there is spillage of blood, pus, urine, vomit or faeces. Therefore, prompt and appropriate disposal of these materials is essential. In all instances the carer must ensure their hands are washed on completion of the task. Whenever dealing with a patient's body fluids it is essential to wear disposable gloves. For information on the correct type of glove, refer to your local policy and comply with universal precautions.

The carer should at all times consider their colleagues and co-workers, who may also be at risk of infection. The laundry staff is at risk from contaminated linen unless the carer has packaged the linen in the correct way.

Activity 9.7

Investigate, using the policy manual as an aid, the correct packaging of the following items:

- Used linen
- Linen soiled with urine and or blood
- Infected linen

Sharps

Accidental inoculation is a minor risk if policies are adhered to, but a major risk if policies are blatantly ignored.

Activity 9.8

Identify your work area's sharps policy and compare this with the actual practice. If there are any discrepancies discuss them with the work area manager.

Remember that the handling of sharps in the clinical area is only the initial part of the process. The portering and disposal will involve a considerable number of personnel who are all at risk of accidental inoculation.

Activity 9.9

Identify what to do if an inoculation injury occurs in your work area.

- To whom is it reported?
- Where is the incident recorded?
- What treatment is the person likely to require?

Some employers offer their employees hepatitis B vaccination via the occupational health department. It is worth enquiring, if you are not already vaccinated.

Waste disposal

The correct disposal of waste from the clinical area is good practice, so it is essential for staff to be fully aware of the relevant policies. Again the carer is only the initial contact in the chain for disposal of waste.

Activity 9.10

Identify the correct containers for the disposal of the following:

- Clinical waste
- General waste
- Aerosols and bottles
- Food waste

Spillage and cleaning

There will be domestic policies for cleaning clinical areas, which by and large will entail damp dusting so as not to create an aerosol effect. Floors will be cleaned with specially designed brooms and machines, to keep air currents to a minimum. Spillages are a hazard to staff and patients and must be dealt with immediately. Small spillages can be wiped up using disposable paper towels. Larger spillages on the floor require mopping. Use clean water and an appropriate detergent to clean the area, then dispose of the water, rinse the utensils and store to enable drying.

Refer to your procedure manual for specific instructions concerning the spillage of blood.

Food handling and hygiene in clinical areas

There is a risk of clients contracting food poisoning if food is not handled safely and in accordance with the Food Safety Act 1990[2]. While the senior person in charge, for example the senior nurse, is responsible for ensuring safe practice is adhered to, each individual carer has a duty of care. The following principles are a guide to safe practice.

Food storage

Food may decompose or become infested or contaminated. Safe storage is therefore essential to minimise this risk in the clinical area:

- Cleanliness: clinical area kitchens should be kept clean, including all storage spaces, especially the refrigerator.
- Cooling: storage below 5 °C in the refrigerator is essential. No food should be stored for more than 24 hours from when it is brought into the area; therefore, it is advisable to date food. Staff food is not to be kept in the same refrigerator. No raw meat, fish, poultry or eggs should be stored in the clients' area. If food is in its original wrapper, only store until the sell by or use by date.
- Regularly check the refrigerator and freezer in a client's home and with their permission dispose of out-of-date items.
- Coverings: all food must be covered and sealed, for example in a re-sealable plastic box. Label the box with the patient's name and the date. Once food has been served, if not consumed, it must be disposed of. Waste bins must be covered at all times with a well-fitting lid.

Food handling

All personnel need to ensure their hands are washed prior to handling and serving meals. A clean disposable plastic apron is ideal to ensure one's clothing does not contaminate the food being handled. Likewise, ensure any cuts or abrasions on your hands are adequately covered. Food should be served at the correct temperature, that is 63 °C or above for hot food, 5 °C or below for cold food, thus reducing the risk of bacterial growth. Re-heating of meals in the clients' area is to be discouraged as it is difficult to ensure that the correct temperature is achieved.

Sample collection

It may be an essential part of the carer's role to collect samples of body fluids for pathology testing to assist in establishing the client's diagnosis. All staff who come into contact with patient's body fluids should wear disposable gloves to reduce the risk of contracting an infection, in particular the human immuno-deficiency virus (HIV), as at the time of writing there is no known vaccine. In addition, the porterage and laboratory staff may be vulnerable if the collection procedure is not adequate.

Ensure the outside of the container is not contaminated during the collection process. If contamination does occur, transfer the contents to a fresh container. Remember, it is not adequate merely to wipe the outside of the container clean, as the microscopic residue will remain. Ensure the lid is securely fastened, insert into a plastic bag and send to pathology in accordance with your local policy. Biohazard labels are recommended to alert staff to the potential hazard[3].

Remember infection is a double-edged situation: you may be at risk of contracting an infection from your work environment or, more likely, your work practice may cause a client to succumb to an infection. The occupational health department can offer a service for monitoring the staff's health status and providing health education. The common cold to you is a nuisance, but to a client it could be a life-threatening chest infection. Cuts or abrasions on your hands offer a port of entry for organisms to establish an infection. To maintain maximum fitness it is necessary to consume a nutritious diet and ensure adequate rest and sleep. Additionally, care of your own clothes and uniform is essential. Adequate separate washing of uniforms at the correct temperature is necessary.

If your employer does not provide a uniform laundry service you may be able to claim the additional laundry costs from the Inland Revenue.

Summary

This chapter has provided a considerable amount of information to enable a better understanding of the modes of spread of organisms. As a carer it is essential to recognise the vulnerability of the sick and ensure safe practices to safeguard them from contracting a hospital-acquired infection. Overall, the single most important consideration in reducing the client's risk is the use of an effective handwashing technique by all carers.

References

1. National Audit Office (2000).
2. Home Office (1990) *Food Safety Act 1990*. HMSO, London.
3. Health Service Advisory Committee (1998) *Safe Working and Prevention of Infection in Clinical Laboratories*. The Stationery Office, London.

Further reading

Docherty, B. (2000) Adopting universal precautions. *Professional Nurse* **15** (6), 358.

King, S. (1998) Decontamination of equipment and the environment. *Nursing Standard* **12** (52), 63–64.

Little, K. (2000) HAI: everybody's business. *Nursing Times* **96** (10), NT Plus.

Pickford, B. (1999) Gunning for the big three. *Nursing Times* **95** (28), 56–58.

Roberts, C. (2000) Universal precautions. *British Journal of Nursing* **9** (1), 43–47.

Royal College of Nursing (2004) *Good Practice in infection control. Guidance for Nursing Staff*. Royal College of Nursing, London.

Royal College of Nursing (2004) *MRSA Guidance for Nursing Staff*. Royal College of Nursing, London.

Salvage, J. (2000) Now wash your hands. *Nursing Times* **96** (43), 22.

Whiller, J. and Cooper, T. (2000) Clean hands; how to encourage good hygiene by patients. *Nursing Times* **96** (46), 37–38.

Chapter 10
Meeting the elimination needs of the client

Christine Ely

Overview

This chapter will consider normal elimination and how psychological, social and cultural influences impact on the client's ability to eliminate waste products from the body. Issues that relate to assisting the client eliminate waste, such as privacy, the equipment required and visual inspection of waste for abnormalities will be explored. Some common problems with elimination, such as constipation, diarrhoea and incontinence will be discussed with strategies to resolve them. The chapter will conclude with consideration of how urinary catheters should be managed and caring for the client who has nausea and vomiting.

Key words: Privacy; dignity; normal elimination; specimens; equipment; elimination problems

Normal elimination

Body processes extract nutrients and energy from food and result in the formation of waste products which must be excreted. Elimination is the term which describes the excretion of waste products, urine and faeces from the body.

Elimination of urine

Chemical waste products are removed from the body cells by the blood which carries this waste to the kidneys. The kidneys are two organs positioned in the upper abdomen at the back (posteriorly) (Fig. 10.1). The blood is filtered by the kidneys and the resulting waste fluid, urine, is passed from the kidneys to be stored in a hollow muscular organ, the bladder. The urine can be voided (emptied) from the body at a convenient time. Voiding of the bladder is called micturition and is controlled by nerve impulses from the brain acting on the muscles.

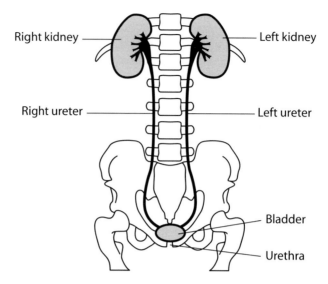

Fig. 10.1 Diagram of the kidneys, bladder and urethra.

Urine is passed from the kidneys to the bladder and is then voided via the urethra. The urethra takes urine from the bladder to outside the body. In men it is about 20 cm (8 inches) long but in women the urethra is shorter, about 3.8 cm (1.5 inches). As the urethra is short, women are more likely to suffer infections, as micro-organisms from outside the body gain easy entry to the urinary tract. Urinary tract infections are called cystitis. The kidneys filter the whole blood volume of an adult, 4–6 litres, 60 times a day. If the kidneys fail to function effectively a person will become fatally ill within a few days as waste toxins build up and they will need treatment with an artificial kidney, or dialysis machine, to stay alive.

Elimination of faeces

Faeces are formed from food waste products in the large bowel (intestine) or colon. This is the lower part of the gastro-intestinal tract, 1.5 m in length, although it is compacted to fit into the abdomen. Normally within the colon are special bacteria (not harmful as long as they stay in the colon) which are essential to complete the breakdown of food. Vitamins B and K are also produced in the colon and any water required by the body is re-absorbed from the faeces back into the blood stream. At the end of the colon is the rectum where faeces accumulate before being expelled from the body via the anus. This process of defecation is normally under voluntary control. Faeces are sometimes referred to as *stools*.

Factors influencing elimination

Elimination is influenced by several factors divided into three categories: psychological, cultural and religious, and social.

Psychological influences

We learn to be independent in using the toilet, or lavatory, when very young. This is an important milestone in a child's life and often merits praise when a child can manage by him- or herself. When clients who have been independent with regard to eliminating have to rely on carers they may suffer embarrassment and even loss of self-esteem. Imagine how you might feel if you had someone wiping your bottom for you. A client may feel helpless like a baby, causing feelings of distress and possible humiliation. In assessing a client's elimination needs, it is important not to appear to treat the adult or child like an infant. It is essential that all those children or adults, who have previously been independent, have their dignity and self-respect preserved[1].

Privacy is very important to the client who needs assistance with elimination, as having to use strange equipment in a different environment may be stressful and embarrassing. Normally we eliminate in private behind closed doors; having to function when only screened by curtains in an area like a ward, with people outside, may make clients feel very uncomfortable. Anxiety about odours and noises might make them put off having to 'go'. Clients' privacy should be ensured, by careful screening with curtains and closing windows, blinds or curtains. Try to avoid interruptions. Imagine what it would feel like to have people walking in on you when you are trying to 'use the toilet'.

Further embarrassment can be caused if clients have to eliminate when meals are being served. The opportunity to use toilet facilities should be offered before meals are served as it can be very unpleasant trying to eat a meal while another client, in the next bed, is using a bedpan or commode. In addition we normally flush away bodily waste without other people having to dispose of it for us. Therefore staff removing a used bedpan or commode may be another source of embarrassment to the client. All bedpans and commodes must be covered with a disposable cover before removal from the bed area. Waste products may have to be examined but this should be done in a dirty utility or sluice area, not at the client's bedside.

Being unable to use normal facilities may cause further anxiety. Adaptations, where necessary, with handrails or raised seats will help the less able to access facilities independently and safely.

Cultural and religious influences

The client may have special names for elimination functions and facilities and accepted practices concerning privacy and post-elimination hygiene. Muslim clients may only use their left hand for wiping themselves. If they cannot use their left hand, they may need help even if their right hand is fully functional. For some people it is not acceptable, whatever their religion, to be assisted with elimination by a carer of the opposite sex. It is important, therefore, to be sensitive to and respect the client's wishes.

Social influences

The type of facilities available in the home environment may influence a client's practices. Those with mobility problems may have adaptations at home or be used to particular equipment. Problems of accessing the toilet may mean the client has to use a commode. Admission to hospital or nursing home may make adjustment to different facilities difficult.

Use of equipment

If clients cannot use the toilet or lavatory, the alternatives are bedpans, commodes or urinals. Before leaving a client on a bedpan or commode the call buzzer must always be within easy reach and toilet paper to hand if he or she can manage on their own.

Activity 10.1

If you have had occasion to have to use a bedpan you will appreciate that they can be difficult and sometimes uncomfortable to use. If you have never experienced sitting on a bedpan, try this to see what it feels like. Share you thoughts about this experience with your colleagues.

Bedpans can be made of either plastic, metal or disposable materials. They should only be used if the client cannot get out of bed to use a commode or be taken to the lavatory. Metal ones can be 'a cold shock' so warming them first (make sure the bedpan is not too hot) is a kindness often much appreciated. Different types of bedpan should be correctly positioned to avoid spillage.

Urinals may be used if the client wishes to pass only urine. Male patients may refer to urinals as 'bottles'. Spills may occur if these overfill and they should be removed for emptying immediately after use and never left on lockers or on the floor where they can look offensive and can easily be knocked over. Specially designed female urinals are available but care is needed when using them to avoid spills. Men often have difficulty in passing urine lying down and may need help to stand by their bed. If necessary the client should be carefully screened and supervised if required.

Commodes must be used with care with brakes applied before the client attempts to sit down. The client on a commode should be positioned near and facing the bed in case they feel faint. The call buzzer must be within easy reach and the client should be instructed to wait for assistance before getting back to bed to avoid falls or accidents. A cover should be used when returning a commode to the sluice or dirty utility area where it should be emptied and cleaned with soap and water or using a specified detergent.

A disposable cover should always be used when taking bedpans, commodes or urinals to or from the client and toilet equipment must always be clean. Bedpans and urinals should be emptied before being placed in the washer to prevent blockages. Before disposing of excreta always be sure that it is not required for inspection, measuring, testing or specimen collection. Bedpans and urinals are normally cleaned in special washers using very hot water at $80\,°C^2$. Care should be taken when removing items from automatic washers as they can be very hot.

It is essential that the carer washes their hands thoroughly after assisting a client to use a bedpan or urinal to prevent the spread of infection. See Chapter 9 for details about infection.

Dealing with unpleasant odours

Clients may have to eliminate in areas where they often eat and spend their days and the odours can be unpleasant and embarrassing. Fresh air dispels odours and aerosol spray is useful. However, sensitivity to client's feelings is important when spraying air freshener as it makes it clear they have caused an offensive smell.

Elimination records

A record of waste elimination – what, when and how much – may be necessary. Fluid balance charts or stool charts may be required for this purpose.

Health and safety

Body waste must be disposed of through the sewage system to ensure that it does not contaminate drinking water supplies, as covered by the Environmental Protection Act 1990 and other waste control legislation[2]. Infections, sometimes with fatal results, can occur if body waste products are not disposed of correctly. Organisational policies must be followed with regard to disposal of waste.

Preventing infection

Good hand washing techniques are essential (see Chapter 9) to prevent cross-infection. Clients must wash their hands after elimination[3]. A bowl of water with soap and towels should be offered at the bedside to clients unable to visit toilet facilities.

Carer's personal clothing

Appropriate protective clothing must be worn when dealing with clients' body waste such as disposable aprons and gloves. Before serving food, disposable aprons, which have been worn when helping clients with elimination, must be changed and hands washed. (Also see Chapter 9.)

Checking for abnormalities

Examination of excreta may reveal abnormalities. Abnormalities detected by visual examination should be reported to the manager/nurse in charge and samples sent to the laboratory for tests if necessary. Therefore, always observe for and report abnormalities before disposing of excreta. This should be done away from the client to avoid embarrassment or causing undue concern. If you are uncertain about what you see, keep the items covered and labelled with the client's name, date and time, in the dirty utility or sluice for inspection by a registered nurse or doctor. Any complaints of soreness, pain or discomfort experienced by the client should be reported as treatment may be required.

Faeces

Colour

This is normally dark brown but abnormal stools may be green with clear mucus, very pale, or fatty in appearance in some bowel disorders. There may be fresh red blood on stools indicating bleeding in the lower intestinal tract (usually the rectum). Bleeding from the upper parts of the intestinal tract, e.g. stomach or duodenum has time to become incorporated into the stools, which therefore look black and tarry with a distinctive smell. However, black tarry stools may also be caused by the client taking iron tablets. Any instance where there is unexplained blood in the stools must be reported to the doctor. Blood in the stools or bleeding from the rectum may be a sign of a serious condition, which will need investigation.

Consistency

Stools should be soft but formed.

Odour

There is often an unpleasant smell, but highly offensive stools do occur in some cases of bowel disease.

Abnormal contents

Parasites or worms may be seen in stools. These are often pale and may be in segments as in the case of tapeworms. Children may swallow small toys and even adults may accidentally swallow tooth caps. However, some adults with mental health problems may deliberately swallow items such as coins.

Urine

Colour

Urine is normally the colour of pale straw. Some medical conditions, drugs and even foods, such as beetroot, can cause the urine to become brightly coloured.

Dark yellow frothy urine can indicate jaundice. If there is an injury to the urinary tract, the urine may be obviously bloodstained. Kidney stones, trauma or cancer in the bladder are some of the problems that may cause bleeding. In women, blood may be present because of menstruation. Blood in the urine is called haematuria and if this occurs it must be reported.

Concentration

This varies according to how much fluid the client drinks. Very dark urine indicates that the client may be dehydrated and not drinking enough. If the client is passing a large quantity of urine, it may become almost clear. This may be because the client has been given drugs called diuretics which remove excessive fluid from the body. Another cause of excess urine production is that the client has a form of diabetes.

Clarity

A cloudy appearance may be a sign of infection. You may observe strands caused by the presence of white blood cells debris due to an infection[4].

Odour

Fresh, normally concentrated, urine has little odour. When the urine is stale it smells of ammonia. If urine has an offensive 'fishy' smell, this indicates an infection in the urinary tract.

Volume

The amount of urine passed in a day is usually dependent on how much the individual drinks. If a person passes less than 200 ml in a 24-hour period, their kidneys may be failing to function effectively. If a person stops passing urine completely this is called anuria; if a person passes large quantities of urine it is called polyuria.

Frequency

Normally urine is passed every 3–4 hours in the daytime. If a client feels that they must pass urine a number of times in an hour then they may have an infection or other medical problem.

Urgency

Urgency is a strong desire to urinate, although the client may not produce any urine when attempting to void. It is usually due to inflammatory lesions in the bladder or urethra or to acute bacterial infections.

Pain or discomfort

If the client has a urinary tract infection they may complain of an intense burning sensation and have the urge to pass urine frequently. Complaints of pain or difficulty when passing urine (dysuria) should be reported.

Urine testing

Abnormalities may not be visible to the naked eye but these can be detected by testing. Urine testing is performed by using reagent 'lab' or 'dip' sticks specially prepared to reveal abnormal constituents when they come in contact with urine (Fig. 10.2). The sticks are dipped into the specimen of urine and colour changes 'read off' to indicate the presence/absence of substances in the urine.

Times when urine may be tested:

- When a client is admitted to hospital or is examined by a doctor; this is often called routine testing and may detect diseases such diabetes mellitus (generally called diabetes), kidney disease or infections of which the client is unaware
- Before a surgical operation

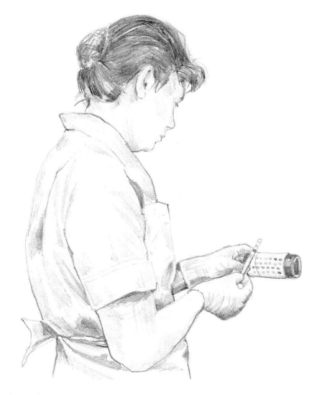

Fig. 10.2 Testing urine.

- If the client is taking certain drugs, which may cause side effects, for example excessive bleeding may occur if the client is taking anti-coagulants
- Clients with diabetes might need regular urine testing but may do this themselves.

If you are asked to obtain a specimen for testing it is important to explain carefully to the client exactly what you require. A clean specimen pot or a jug (only used for urine) should be used. It should be labelled with the client's name or a cover with the client's name may be used. This is important to ensure that specimens are not muddled.

Procedure for testing urine, using reagent strips:

1. Urine must be tested when it is fresh as urine alters with the passage of time and this can give false results.
2. Ensure that your hands are clean and dry. It is advisable to wear disposable gloves.
3. Only use reagent containers that have been kept closed. Moisture in the air causes the sticks to deteriorate, often in about 20 minutes.
4. Check the expiry date on the reagent strip container, as out-of-date strips will give false results.
5. Remove a stick carefully and replace the lid immediately. **Do not touch the coloured squares of the stick or put the stick down** as moisture from seemingly dry hands or other surfaces can give false results.
6. The stick should be dipped into the urine, removed, then tapped lightly on the rim of the container to remove excess urine. Note the exact time that you do this.
7. Wait for the exact time stated in the instructions and immediately compare the results of any colour change on the stick with the guide on the reagent container. If the stick is left for longer that the recommended time misleading results may occur. Be careful not to allow the stick to touch the side of the container.
8. Note the results, write these on the client's records and inform the nurse or doctor.

The results – what do they mean?

pH

This means how acid or alkaline the urine is (7 is neutral). A figure below 7 is acid and above is alkaline. Normal urine is in the range of between 5 and 8. Vegetarians usually have urine that is more alkaline – around pH 8.

Blood or haemoglobin

Although it may not look as if blood is present in the urine, there may be a positive reaction. Blood in urine can be caused by trauma, menstruation in women, or other bladder conditions. Some drugs may cause bleeding in the urinary tract.

Glucose

The presence of glucose or sugar could indicate diabetes. However, more tests would be required to confirm this.

Ketones

These occur as the result of the body breaking down fats to produce energy when it cannot use sugars, for example, in clients with untreated diabetes or in the client who is fasting or in cases of starvation.

Urobilinogen and bilirubin

These are abnormalities associated with liver problems.

Protein

This occurs in infections and where there has been kidney damage, or as a complication of pregnancy.

Specific gravity

This indicates how concentrated the urine is but is not always measured. The normal range of specific gravity is 1004–1040.

Specimen collection

Further tests may be required on the client's excreta and specimens must be collected in special pots/containers. Specimens must be clearly labelled with the client's name, registration number, and the date and time the specimen was obtained. Containers must be placed in plastic bags (to prevent infection) with a written request form completed by the doctor. Specimens must be dispatched to the laboratory as soon as possible. If they cannot be sent immediately, they may need to be stored in a special specimen refrigerator. Specimens must never be kept in the same refrigerator as food or medicines.

Stool specimens

This type of specimen may be required if infection is suspected or for blood that is not visible (occult blood). Parasites may need to be clearly identified. Occasionally specimen collection may be required over a period of days for which special large containers are needed.

Urine specimens

Some urine specimens may need to be collected in a specific way to ensure that they are not contaminated.

Mid-stream specimen of urine (MSU)

This specimen is tested to correctly identify organisms causing a suspected infection of the urinary tract so that the correct antibiotic or other treatment can be prescribed. The first part of the urine stream is discarded as it may contain contaminated cells from the urethra. A mid-stream sample is then collected in the specimen pot. Instructions to the client need to be given carefully and clearly – following organisational policy. This is rather a complicated procedure for someone doing it for the first time.

(1)   The client must be instructed not to touch the inside of the specimen pot or the underside of the lid as this will contaminate the specimen.
(2)   The client should clean around the urethral opening with cotton wool and sterile saline solution.
(3)   The client should pass a small amount of urine into the toilet and then stop and pass some urine into the specimen pot.
(4)   If they still need to pass any more urine, this can be done into the toilet.

Early morning specimen of urine (EMSU)

This specimen is collected from the first urine the client passes on waking in the morning. The urine is most concentrated on waking and this type of specimen may be required when abnormal cells are suspected.

24-hour collection of urine

The total volume of urine passed in a 24-hour period is collected. A starting time is identified and the client asked to pass urine; normally the first urine passed on waking in the morning. This is discarded but from this point onward for 24 hours all the urine passed is retained in large plastic containers. The containers may have special preservatives added so care must be taken not to spill any contents. A 24-hour collection may be needed to determine kidney function or hormone levels. Should urine be discarded accidentally this should be reported immediately as a new collection will have to be made.

Catheter specimen of urine (CSU)

If a client has an indwelling catheter a urine specimen is collected from a special port on the tube of the catheter. This may be done with a sterile syringe and needle and great care must be taken to ensure that no contamination of the catheter system occurs. Specimens should never be taken from the catheter drainage bag.

A final note about specimens

Although you may become used to collecting excreta, clients and their visitors may not be used to seeing it. Specimens for dispatch to the laboratory should be placed away from the public gaze and not on top of lockers, cupboards or desks.

Constipation

Normal faeces are semi-formed and soft. This makes the passage easy through the anus. If the consistency of the stool changes and it becomes hard and dry it will be difficult to pass and the client may experience discomfort and even pain when having a bowel action. The client may not be able to open their bowels as often as usual for them and this infrequency and difficulty is called constipation. It is important that constipation is prevented as it can lead to faecal incontinence[5].

Causes of constipation

Changes in activity, the environment, diet or medication can all result in constipation. It is a common problem when clients experience a change in lifestyle brought about by either moving into a nursing home or admission to hospital. Loss of appetite due to illness and disinclination to drink, which often occurs in elderly people whose thirst reflexes have declined with advancing age, can lead to constipation. Lack of fresh air and exercise, reduced mobility and the difficulty of not being able to use the facilities when the client experiences the urge 'to go' can all contribute to constipation. Clients who are depressed are not only likely to be less mobile, they may lack the motivation to follow an appropriate diet[6].

Some drugs, especially strong pain killing (analgesic) preparations such as morphine or other opiates may cause constipation as well as iron supplements, calcium, some antacids, anti-histamines and anti-depressants. Although constipation is rarely life-threatening it can cause misery and discomfort[7]. Constipation can, however, cause confusion in the elderly and changes in bowel habit that cannot be easily explained should be investigated as this may indicate a serious condition.

Treatments for constipation

Diet

Activity 10.2

List some foods which you know can prevent constipation.

Your answer might include:

- Fruit such as apples, oranges and bananas
- Bran and whole wheat cereals
- Brown rice
- Wholewheat pasta
- Drinking plenty of fluids (not alcohol)
- Wholewheat bread
- Vegetables

Diets that contain roughage or fibre and plenty of fluids, usually at least 2–3 litres a day, are needed to prevent constipation. Action should always be taken to improve the diet, if possible, before any other forms of treatment, as this is the natural way to resolve constipation. The older client may need particular guidance with regard to including sufficient fibre in the diet[8]. Exercise should be encouraged to prevent constipation.

Laxatives

Laxatives soften the stool, add bulk, or stimulate the gut wall into increased activity. These substances may be useful but even bulk laxatives like bran may have side effects such as feelings of abdominal discomfort and flatulence[9]. They should only be used for exceptional instances not on a regular basis as laxative abuse causes damage to the bowel and long-term over-use can cause faecal incontinence. Clients should be referred to their doctors for advice about regular use of laxatives as, in general, this should be avoided. If laxatives are ineffective other measures may be required.

Suppositories

These are semi-solid pellets, e.g. glycerine suppositories, which soften the stool to make its passage easier. One or two of these are inserted into the rectum and allowed to dissolve. Medicines, which are not aimed at causing the client to open their bowels can also be given in suppository form, as drugs can be absorbed into the bloodstream through the bowel wall. This can be useful if the client is vomiting and cannot absorb the drug through the stomach.

Enemas

Enemas are warm water or specially prepared solutions which are introduced into the rectum to stimulate the bowel to empty. Medication can also be given in enema form.

Suppositories and enemas should be prescribed and should only be given by specially trained staff. Inserting any object into the rectum is potentially hazardous as the bowel wall may rupture.

Positioning clients for suppositories and enemas

The bedclothes should be protected with incontinence pads and the client should be place on their left side with knees drawn up towards the chin. The client should be covered as much as possible.

Impacted faeces and manual removal

Faeces which are so hard that they cannot be passed at all are called 'impacted'. An enema of oil may be given to soften the faeces and then these may be removed

using a gloved hand. Normally only a registered nurse or doctor should undertake this procedure because it is painful and hazardous.

Privacy, dignity and consent

These treatments can be very uncomfortable and distressing. It is important that
the client is correctly positioned and not exposed. Dignity[1] should be preserved
and privacy is essential. The client must consent to any such treatment[10], otherwise this can be considered an assault. The client should be supported during
such procedures and commodes and bedpans must be readily at hand as the
client may feel a sudden and uncontrollable urge to open their bowels.

Diarrhoea

Most people have experienced diarrhoea at some time in their lives. This is the
passage of watery or unformed stools often at frequent intervals and accompanied by abdominal pain and discomfort. The anus may become very sore from
frequent evacuations.

Activity 10.3

Make a list of some causes of diarrhoea which you know.

Your list may include:

- Stressful events as these may disturb normal bowel function
- Infections of the gut such as salmonella (food poisoning), which may occur
  on foreign holidays
- Intolerance of foods and milk feeds
- Antibiotics, which may cause diarrhoea as they destroy protective bacteria
  normally present in the colon and when these are absent other organisms
  can flourish and cause infections
- Severe constipation with faecal impaction, which may result in diarrhoea
  leaking around the obstruction; this is called 'impaction with overflow'

Treatment

If an infection is suspected a specimen of stool will be required for laboratory
analysis. Great care must be taken with bowel infections as they spread very
rapidly and can even be fatal in vulnerable clients such as young children and
older people. Clients with diarrhoea are often nursed in isolation (barrier
nursing) to prevent spread of the condition. Organisational policies should be
followed in cases of such infections. Medications may be given to alleviate diarrhoea. Both the carer and the client should strictly adhere to hygeine and hand-

washing routines to prevent cross-infection. (See Chapter 9 for details of handwashing.)

Urinary and faecal incontinence

This is the inability to control urinary or faecal elimination after normal control has been established in infancy. Incontinence may affect older children and adults. It is a problem often associated with old age although it is wrong to think that nothing can be done to treat incontinence in older people. The term incontinence has many negative connotations and 'loss of control' may be a preferable term to prevent a client being labelled incontinent[11]. Specially trained nurses, often called continence advisers, should be contacted to assess a client and offer specialist advice concerning treatments and equipment. Clients in the community may need special services, e.g. delivery of equipment and disposal of waste.

> As men draw near the common goal
> Can anything be sadder?
> That master of his soul
> Is servant to his bladder.
> (Anonymous[12])

Causes of incontinence

- Muscle weakness of the pelvic floor muscles results in urinary incontinence. This is often related to child-bearing in women, and sometimes occurs when mothers are not encouraged to persist with post-natal exercises.
- Obstruction of the urethra, which may occur in men owing to enlargement of the prostate gland.
- Obesity, where excessive soft tissue in the abdomen causes pressure on the bladder[13].
- Nerve damage to nerve pathways which regulate bladder function[14], for example after spinal injury.
- Clients with severe learning difficulties.
- Emotional causes such as severe anxiety.
- 'Confusion' which may be associated with acute illness, e.g. high fever or long term in cases of dementia.
- 'Institutional' where clients in long-term care homes have become lethargic and dependent on carers with negative attitudes, who do not actively manage incontinence.
- Older people need to empty their bladders more frequently as the capacity declines with age[15].
- Clients who have had strokes often also have urinary incontinence[16].
- Clients who have conditions leading to frequency and/or urgency usually associated with urinary infections or inflammation of the tract (see section on Checking for abnormalities, p. 130).

Psychological and social effects of incontinence

Incontinence is a condition present when a person loses control of bladder or bowel function and passes urine or faeces at socially inappropriate times or places. Babies who have not acquired control of their elimination functions are 'allowed' to soil themselves but soon after children learn to walk they are encouraged to become 'toilet trained'. Incontinence then becomes a source of embarrassment and humiliation as the child grows older. Bedwetting (enuresis) in children can be as much a psychological problem as a physical one and should not be ignored[17]. Adult incontinence is likely to lead to social isolation in that they do not want to mix with other people and fear going out in case an 'accident occurs' and there is also great concern about soiling and distressing odours in public.

Incontinence is often associated with those of advancing age and those who are disabled but it can occur at any age. Sometimes little can be done to cure the problem, for example, where there is nerve damage to the spine, severe dementia, or in those who are terminally ill and unconscious. However, in some cases, treatments can improve the situation and in all cases strategies can be used to minimise the distressing effects of incontinence. Therefore, a positive attitude towards managing incontinence is essential. Faecal incontinence may be very embarrassing and clients may avoid seeking help[18].

Urinary incontinence in women is often associated with trauma following childbirth and may become worse later in life. Some women may feel unclean and this may affect sexual relationships or those of some religious groups, such as Muslims, may not feel able to pray as they feel unclean[19].

Stress incontinence

This occurs when clients experience incontinence when they laugh, cough or sneeze. The weakness of the pelvic floor muscles causes small amounts of urine to be passed when abdominal pressure increases. Clients may fear social occasions due to the humiliation of wetting yourself in public. Exercise or electrical stimulation treatment given by physiotherapists can improve muscle tone but corrective surgery may be required to repair the damage.

Incontinence caused by medications

Clients may have been prescribed drugs such as diuretics to make them pass urine because they retain too much fluid in their bodies, and they may suddenly need to use bedpans, commodes or go to the toilet. It is well to be aware of this in advance as the client may not have the ability to control him/herself once the drugs act. Therefore, being prepared with equipment ready at the bedside or being positioned within easy reach of toilet facilities may prevent temporary incontinence. If clients are treated with laxatives, suppositories or enemas they may experience similar urgency to defecate and again anticipation and preparation may prevent incontinence and embarrassment.

Preventing and managing incontinence

Managing incontinence is about ensuring that the client can use facilities. Factors need to be assessed carefully and measures taken to remove difficulties in accessing toilet facilities. Carers should be alert to difficulties and report these to ensure that corrective steps are taken.

- Mobility – Can the client get to the toilet? Poor footwear, swollen feet or toenail problems can reduce mobility and indirectly cause incontinence. If clients have been unwell and are beginning to mobilise they should not start this by walking to the toilet. Initially they should be taken in a wheelchair and then should walk back in their own time. They may be anxious about getting to the toilet and falls can result from rushing to get there in time.
- Distance to the toilet – If this is too far incontinence may result
- Eyesight – Can they see when using the facilities and is lighting adequate?
- Dexterity – Can they remove clothing in time? Should their clothing be adapted?
- Confusion – Do they know when to go? If confusion is the case the client may need reminding and be guided to the toilet at regular intervals. After a period of illness, older individuals may need 're-training'.
- Equipment – Toilets should be adapted with rails and raised seats so that clients can use facilities independently.

Carers' attitudes and clients' feelings

The effects of incontinence may be wide-ranging – complete loss of control or minimal soiling and/or dribbling of urine. Clients must never be blamed for incontinence. When clients are embarrassed and upset by their incontinence carers may wish to reassure them, but we must be careful when using simple phrases like 'We don't mind', 'We are used to it' or 'It doesn't matter, we don't have to wash the sheets' as although such remarks are meant to be well meaning they may not allow the client to express *their* feelings. Reassurance that you can deal with the problem is important but let the client say how they feel first. Remember, although it may not matter to you it does matter to them. When cleaning clients who have been incontinent ensure that dignity and privacy are not compromised.

Confused clients

If clients do not know when they need to go to the toilet then they should be taken at regular intervals. A special regimen may be necessary so this is achieved but it might be advisable not to walk the client about at night-time when a commode can be used instead.

Soiled linen and clothing

Linen soiled with client's excreta needs to be dealt with separately from linen that is just dirty. Most organisations have special bags which dissolve in the large linen cleaning machines without laundry staff having to unwrap the bags. In hospitals or care homes if clients' own clothes are soiled they should be placed in plastic bags and dispatched to personal laundry facilities or relatives informed as soon as possible so that items can be removed for cleaning. (For personal cleansing for incontinent clients see Chapter 11.)

Pads and protective clothing

A wide range of protective clothing and pads can be offered to the client. However, expert advice should be sought and assessment by a continence adviser will ensure that appropriate protection is given[20]. The client may also need support when initially given protective clothing to wear as the notion of wearing something akin to a nappy can be distressing. The client may be embarrassed about buying such aids and may choose sanitary pads instead but these are not always suitable for use with urinary or faecal incontinence. Client choice is important when selecting products[21]. Pads should be changed regularly and clients kept clean; used pads must be placed in a disposal bag or bin and never placed on the bathroom or toilet floor. Used pads and incontinence sheets should be disposed of according to the organisation's policy. At home a special service for delivery and collection of pads may be necessary.

Urinary catheters

A urinary catheter is used when the client is unable either to pass or control their flow of urine. They can be used as a temporary measure or in some circumstances be needed for long-term care.

A urinary catheter is a plastic tube used for drainage of the bladder (Fig. 10.3). They are usually flexible tubes, the diameter of a pen, 45 cm in length for men and 25 cm for women, with a small inflatable balloon at the tip just below the drainage eyelet. The tube is sterile and is passed into the bladder using aseptic technique to prevent the spread of infection. The balloon is inflated with sterile

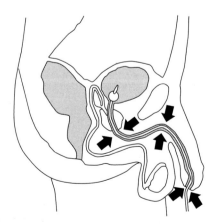

Fig. 10.3   The bladder with a self-retaining catheter in position.

water, not air, to provide weight to keep the catheter in position. The catheter is connected to a drainage bag and this provides a closed system which will allow urine to empty from the bladder but should prevent infections occurring.

The system seems such a simple way of dealing with incontinence that you may wonder why it is not used more widely for those who cannot control bladder function. However, there are problems, as even with the greatest care infection can occur and this may be very serious as clients can die from urinary tract infections. The catheter can become blocked with mucus, its very presence can be irritating and having urine draining into a bag, possibly visible to others, can result in a negative effect on self-esteem.

Therefore, the decision to catheterise should only be taken following careful assessment. There may be other treatments for incontinence that should be considered first. However, there are situations where the decision to pass a catheter is most appropriate, e.g. a client unable to pass urine due to blockage, serious illness when specific measures of urinary function are required, following surgery, or where the client has long-term problems unlikely to improve such as multiple sclerosis. Urinary catheters can therefore either be left in position (indwelling) or may be passed when the bladder is full and needs emptying (intermittent catheterisation).

Preventing infection and maintaining function

If a urinary catheter is passed care to prevent infection must be immaculate. Whenever a problem occurs not only should it be dealt with but consideration needs to be given to the reason why this occurred and how to prevent it happening again[22]. This means that if you notice anything abnormal about the client's catheter you should report it so that preventive action can be taken to ensure correct function. Maintaining good intake of oral fluids for clients with catheters can significantly reduce blockage, but asking an older person to drink between 2 litres and 3 litres of fluid a day is sometimes difficult. For this reason, careful explanations need to be given to older clients about catheter care.

Keeping urinary catheters clean

The area where the catheter enters the body must be kept clean to avoid micro-organisms entering the urinary tract. Normally inside the bladder is a sterile environment (with no micro-organisms), this means there are no defensive mechanisms, unlike the colon where bowel bacteria can help prevent infections (see Chapter 9). Therefore, to keep micro-organisms out, clean the catheter tubing outside the body by wiping down the tube away from the client. The plan of care will contain instructions of the cleaning materials to be used, usually sterile normal saline with sterile gauze swabs or non-perfumed soap and water. Observation should be made for signs of discharge around the catheter where it enters the client's body, and a check made for leakage of urine, which can occur if the catheter is the wrong size. Any discharge or leakage should be reported promptly.

Keeping the catheter secure

Pulling on the catheter will cause pain and discomfort. This can be avoided if the catheter is carefully secured to the client's leg using tape, but this should not be too tight. Never pin catheters to bedclothes as this restricts movement and can cause trauma. The tubing must not become twisted or kinked or it will fail to drain. If the drainage bag should need to be lifted up, urine must not be allowed to siphon (drain) back into the client, therefore folding the tubing or pinching it with the fingers can prevent back flow. Clamps are sometimes used but are potentially hazardous as they may be forgotten and cause obstruction. The drainage bag should not be dragged on the floor, as this will increase the likelihood of infection. The bag should be attached to a special stand and the exit port at the bottom of the bag must be off the floor. Special bags which can be strapped to the client's leg are preferable to clients walking around carrying their urine bags.

The drainage bag should be emptied at regular intervals, usually at least three times a day or to fit in with the client's personal routine. Disposable gloves should be worn for this procedure. Prior to opening, the drainage port may be cleaned with a spirit swab in line with the organisation's prevention of infection policy. Care must be taken when opening and closing the drainage port to prevent contamination. The urine should be drained into an appropriate container, such as a large plastic jug, used only for this purpose. The drainage bag should be changed when required but disconnecting the catheter and reconnecting to a new bag should be done with great care, as this is another potential source of contamination.

Removal of indwelling catheters

When removing an indwelling catheter you should have ready a disposable bag for clinical waste and a syringe to remove the water in the balloon. Disposable gloves should be worn and a disposable towel should protect the clothing and/or bedclothes. The syringe is attached to the balloon part to withdraw the water (check that the correct amount of water is removed) and when the balloon is deflated the catheter can be gently removed and immediately placed in the disposable bag. Inspect the catheter to ensure it is complete.

Intermittent catheterisation

Some clients may pass a catheter themselves which is removed when the urine has drained from the bladder. This means that there is less chance of causing infection[23] and the client does not have to wear a bag device. Clients in the community who have conditions such as spina bifida or multiple sclerosis may use this form of catheterisation.

Penile sheaths for male clients

These are like condoms with a tube attached at the tip which can drain into a catheter drainage bag. They are less likely to cause infection than a catheter but irritation can sometimes occur and they should only be used following careful assessment of the client and his problem.

Colostomy

A colostomy or stoma is an opening of the colon (large bowel) on to the surface of the abdomen. Faeces can then pass out of this opening into a disposable plastic bag or dressing applied to the stoma. The stoma is created surgically to relieve obstruction due to disease or more commonly cancer of the bowel. The colostomy may be temporary or permanent. Special care of the skin area round the stoma is required and advice about this and the management of the stoma can be obtained from specialist stoma care nurses.

Ileostomy

This is similar to a colostomy but the opening is made into the small bowel. The faecal discharge is therefore much more fluid and contains digestive enzymes which are destructive to the skin. The stoma is spout shaped so that it can be safely tucked inside a bag attached to the skin surface and thus fluid discharge is prevented from making contact with skin. Careful application of drainage bags and meticulous skin care are essential.

Haemorrhoids (piles)

These are grossly enlarged (varicose) veins of the anal canal. They may be inside or outside the body. If seen from the outside they have the appearance of a bunch of small grapes. Haemorrhoids can bleed if damaged and be very painful and itchy. They can result from straining due to constipation, obesity and pregnancy – all conditions which raise abdominal pressure. Treatments for haemorrhoids include special creams and suppositories, or in severe cases, surgery may be required.

Nausea and vomiting

Normally food is eaten then digested. However, if normal function of the stomach is disturbed because of illness, the contents of the stomach may be forcefully expelled and vomited. The sensation of wanting to vomit is called nausea and this may be associated with various problems of the gastro-intestinal tract or be caused by drugs or anxiety. The after-effects of anaesthetic gases used during surgery may also make the client feel nauseated and even vomit. Therefore, a vomit bowl should always be at the bedside following operation. Vomiting can be prevented with drugs, and therefore nausea should be reported so that appropriate medication can be administered[24].

Problems caused by nausea and vomiting

- Loss of fluid and electrolytes
- Medicines not fully absorbed before vomiting
- Soreness and unpleasant taste in the mouth caused by acid from the stomach
- Feelings of exhaustion and distress
- Other clients or onlookers may be distressed and become nauseated themselves

Inhaled vomit which enters the lungs causes serious complications which may be life-threatening. The airway may become blocked or vomit may enter the lungs and cause a virulent form of pneumonia which is difficult to treat. Clients who are vomiting must never be left unattended.

Action to take following a client vomiting

1. Protect or screen from general view.
2. Support the person in an upright position or roll onto the side to prevent vomit inhalation.
3. Offer mouthwashes or opportunity to clean teeth with a toothbrush.
4. The vomit must be inspected prior to disposal to note how much fluid has been lost and the nature of the content, e.g. any unabsorbed tablets or undigested food.
5. Details may need to be entered on a fluid chart, especially if the vomiting is repeated.

Vomiting blood

In some conditions, clients may vomit either fresh or partially digested blood. The medical term for vomiting blood is haematemesis. This can occur because blood has been swallowed from trauma to the mouth (then vomited), or bleeding from the stomach or oesophagus. Vomiting blood can be very frightening for the client and if a large amount of blood is lost the client may collapse – this is a medical emergency.

Summary

The removal of body waste is an essential activity of daily living. For those clients who are unable to meet their elimination needs unaided it is important that carers maintain dignity and self-esteem as well as promote independence.

References

1. Human Rights Act (1998) European Convention of Human Rights, Articles 3 and 8. Available at www.echr.coe.int (accessed on 20/09/03).

2. Rogers, R., Salvage, J. and Cowell, R. (1999) *Nurses at Risk. A Guide to Health and Safety at Work*, 2nd edition. Macmillan, Basingstoke.

3. Whiller, J. and Cooper, T. (2000) Clean hands: how to encourage good hygiene by patients. *Nursing Times* **96** (46), 37–38.

4. Skinner, S. (1996) *Understanding Clinical Investigations*. Bailliere Tindall, London.

5. Brocklehurst, J., Dickenson, E. and Winsor, J. (1999) Laxatives and faecal incontinence in long-term care. *Nursing Standard* **13** (52), 32–36.

6. Vickery, G. (1997) Basics of constipation. *Gastroenterology Nursing* **20** (4), 125–128.

7. Winney, J. (1998) Constipation. *Nursing Standard* **13** (11), 49–56.

8. Wheatley, F. (2000) All bunged up. *Nursing Standard* **14** (40), 27.

9. Day, A. (2001) The nurse's role in managing constipation. *Nursing Standard* **16** (8), 41–44.

10. Addison, R., Ness, W. and Abulafi, M. (2000) How to administer enemas and suppositories. *Nursing Times NT Plus: Continence* **96** (6), 3–4.

11. Thomas, S. (2000) Continence in older people: a priority for primary care. *Nursing Standard* **15** (25), 45–50.

12. Anonymous (1938) *The Speculum, Melbourne* No. 140.

13. Johnson, S.T. (2000) From incontinence to confidence. *Americal Journal of Nursing* **100** (2), 69–75.

14. Bardsley, A. (2000) The neurogenic bladder. *Nursing Standard* **14** (22), 39–41.

15. Sander, R. (1999) Promoting urinary continence in residential care. *Nursing Standard* **14** (13–15), 49–53.

16. Brittain, K. (2001) Stroke and continence care. *Nursing Times* **97** (30), 57.

17. Rogers, J. (1998) Nocturnal enuresis should not be ignored. *Nursing Standard* **13** (9), 35–38.

18. Norton, C. (1997) Faecal incontinence in adults *Nursing Standard* **11** (46), 49–56.

19. Wilkinson, K. (2001) Pakistani women's perceptions and experiences of incontinence. *Nursing Standard* **16** (5), 33–39.

20. Morrison, C. (2001) Disposable body-worn pads for incontinence. *Nursing Times* **97** (30NT Plus), 58–59.

21. White, H. (2001) Continence products in the community: towards a more client-centred service. *Professional Care of Mother and Child* **11** (4), 105–107.

22. Simpson, L. (2001) Indwelling urethral catheters. *Nursing Standard* **15** (46), 47–53.

23. Barton, R. (2000) Intermittent self-catheterisation. *Nursing Standard* **15** (9), 47–52.

24. Jolley, S. (2001) Managing post-operative naurea and vomiting. *Nursing Standard* **15** (4), 47–53.

Further reading

Getliffe, K. (1996) Care of urinary catheters. *Nursing Standard* **11** (11), 47–54.

May, H. (1998) Now wash your hands. *Nursing Times* **94** (4), 63–66.

Roper, N., Logan, W. and Tierney, A.J. (1996) *The Elements of Nursing*, 4th edition. Churchill Livingstone, Edinburgh.

Sneddon, D. (1999) Continence assessment in long-term care. *Professional Nurse* **15** (1), 32–34.

Spencer, G. (1999) The role of exercise in successful ageing. *Professional Nurse* **15** (2), 105–108.

Chapter 11
Meeting the hygiene needs of the client

Christine Ely

Overview

This chapter explores issues related to personal hygiene. Psychological, cultural and social influences are considered. It is also important that carers understand issues of privacy, consent and dignity. The normal function of the skin is explained and possible abnormalities outlined. The processes involved in meeting clients' hygiene needs are described to ensure comfort and safety are preserved and the topics include body image, use of skin products, shaving and mouth and eye care. The chapter concludes with an overview of dealing with skin infestations.

Key words: Hygiene; consent; privacy; dependency; social interaction; body image; mouth care; cosmetics; infestations

Influences on hygiene

Personal hygiene is concerned with care of the skin, hair, eyes and mouth. Good standards of personal hygiene are essential. The Department of Health (2001) states that the desired outcome when meeting a client's personal and oral hygiene needs are that:

> clients are clean, comfortable and their appearance maintained according to their personal preference and religious/cultural needs . . . clients' mouths are clean and optimum comfort and function are maintained.
>
> (Department of Health 2001, p. 52[1])

Factors influencing hygiene practices

Daily washing and bathing routines are very personal but are influenced by a number of factors (Fig. 11.1).

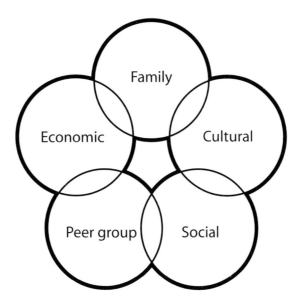

Fig. 11.1   Factors influencing hygiene practices.

Family

We start our lives by being washed by our guardians, usually mothers, and many people continue childhood routines into adult life, such as cleaning teeth in the morning and evening. Family habits vary with regard to bathing in the morning or evening.

Economic

Bathrooms as we know them are comparatively new; they were not standard in many homes in the UK until after the 1930s. The cost of heating water may concern some clients making them less inclined to bath and to prefer 'a good wash'.

Social isolation

Those who have very little contact with others either by choice or because of personal circumstances, for example older clients, those with disabilities or those who are housebound may be less motivated to pay attention to personal hygiene. Clients with disorders such as depression may lose interest in their personal appearance and not feel like bothering to wash. Personal neglect may be a sign of deteriorating mental health.

Cultural influences and differences

Attitudes to washing may vary between cultural and religious groups. Some may have strict practices and taboos. In many Western countries strong body odour is considered offensive (sales of deodorants are a testimony to this) while in other countries body odour is normal and socially acceptable. In some religions, high value is placed on personal cleanliness as it is linked to spiritual renewal.

Clients' choice

When deciding how often clients need to wash, a balance needs to be achieved between their medical condition, the desire to promote health through cleanliness, and the need to respect their rights to make an informed choice about their own personal hygiene routines. Although changing poor hygiene practices by adapting routines to improve health and prevent infection may be encouraged, the issue should be handled with sensitivity and not forced. However, it has to be remembered that in institutions where clients have to live in close contact and share communal facilities, poor hygiene practices may cause others offence or harm.

Consent

It is essential that carers appreciate that if clients are forced to bath or be bathed against their will, the carers could be considered to be committing an offence. Touching someone against their will can be considered a trespass on their person. In the UK, clients can never be forced to have a treatment against their will and even if he or she has a mental health problem they may still be deemed competent to decide to refuse an intervention[2]. Therefore, if a client adamantly refuses to be bathed this must be respected. Prior to meeting hygiene needs the client's consent should always be obtained. An explanation should be given and permission obtained from the client to have this done to them. If clients do not obviously refuse and appear to be compliant, it may be assumed that consent is implied. However, if clients in any way object or, for example, refuse to allow you to undress them, you must not continue to try to remove their clothes. At this point, you should listen carefully to the reason *why* the client does not wish you to proceed. Advice should be immediately sought from the registered nurse if you are unable to obtain consent and the client does not wish to co-operate in the care that you have been directed to offer.

Nakedness and privacy

Today some people expose more of their bodies than did previous generations. Many of today's older people rarely undressed in front of others, even their spouses. Personal hygiene was achieved by removing items of clothing separately and washing one part of the body at a time. Those over 80 years may have memories of washing in a tin bath in front of the fire as many houses of working people had no bathrooms in those days. Modesty as demonstrated by keeping the body covered is valued by some religious groups, especially among women, for example, strict Muslims. They may also have taboos concerning being washed by a carer of the opposite sex.

In some institutions there may be communal wash areas although less so nowadays, and though some clients may not be embarrassed when washing or shaving in front of others, it is always important to consider the issue of privacy and to remember that clients have a legal right to privacy[3].

Protecting privacy of clients in institutions

- Bed areas must be fully screened with no gaps between curtains.
- Staff should respect privacy and avoid intruding by unnecessarily opening curtains when clients may be exposed.
- Window blinds should be drawn as clients may be overlooked.
- Always knock before entering bathrooms.

Feeling dependent

Young children and babies need to be bathed and part of growing up is learning how to care for your own body. As adults we are normally fully able to wash ourselves. Having this done for you is perhaps something you might not have experienced in your adult life.

Activity 11.1

What is it like to washed? With a friend or partner, wash each other's hands and faces. This is best done blindfold to test your communication skills as well. Afterwards give each other feedback. Was the water temperature right and was your partner gentle enough? Be truthful and share with each other what it was really like.

Activity 11.1 will have given you some insight into how a client who has to be washed all over might feel. You may have felt a bit like a baby. Some clients feel very distressed at regressing or returning to a childlike state. This can be especially distressing if recovery of full independence is unlikely. The use of a sensible approach is important but the carer should not assume a mother-like role as this might discourage a client who is able to regain their independence.

Social interaction: a time to talk

Assisting clients with meeting their hygiene needs creates an opportunity for the client and the carer to talk privately. Clients who are worried or anxious may feel more comfortable about asking difficult questions or disclosing concerns when the curtains are drawn or in the security of a locked bathroom. Clients should be allowed time and opportunity to express themselves and carers should be supportive and prepared to listen to the client's worries. Carers' should report any significant issues to the registered nurse and the client should be reassured that 'confidentiality of information' will be respected within the care team.

The carer's personal clothing

Plastic aprons, as protective clothing, should always be worn when washing clients and these must be changed prior to serving food. It is normally unnecessary to wear disposable gloves except when cleaning the buttocks and genital areas. Advice should be sought when washing patients who are being nursed with special infection control precautions.

How hygiene needs should be met – the care plan

If the client has a perceived problem in meeting their hygiene needs, this will be included in the client's care plan devised by the registered nurse. Clients may be totally dependent or only require minimal assistance. Supervision rather than actual 'hands on' help may be all that is needed as in the case of some clients with mental health problems. The degree of help required may alter as the client's condition changes.

The care plan should indicate the following:

- What level of independence is realistically to be aimed for, within a given time, so that your client will be working towards achievable goals? Some clients will always need some help while others will quickly regain their former level of independence.
- Which areas are to be cleaned and how? Clients may have problems using soap and aqueous cream may be used instead or specific prescribed lotions may need to be applied.
- If appropriate, which areas must not be washed? (For example, skin markings where a client is receiving radiotherapy or operation sites.)

Body image

The term body image refers to, as it suggests, the mental picture we have of ourselves. It concerns our sexuality, that is, the way we express our sexual orientation (see Chapter 3).

Activity 11.2

Consider how you imagine you look. Do others always confirm this image?
Also have you ever looked at a photograph of yourself and said 'Is that me?' or 'Do I really look like that!'
Are you particularly conscious of any of your features?

So, why do we not always recognise ourselves? Is it that our body image is not quite the same as reality? An exaggerated example of this is the mental health disorder anorexia nervosa when the sufferer has a distorted image of himself or herself as a very fat person, when in fact they are abnormally thin.

Activity 11.3

Make a list of conditions or situations which may affect a client's body image.

You might have included:

- Scarring
- Loss of a limb (amputation)
- Removal of a breast (mastectomy)
- Skin disorders
- Weight loss
- Hair loss
- Stoma such as colostomy or ileostomy
- Paralysis of a limb (hemiplegia) as caused by a stroke
- Damage due to wounds or burns
- Clients with dementia who may not recognise themselves

When assisting with hygiene needs, carers need to be aware that the sight of their altered body may distress a client. The client may be embarrassed and expect a negative response on the part of the carer. It is important not to give this impression by non-verbal signs. Carers should be supportive, allowing the client to express their feelings, as this will assist the eventual acceptance of a changed body image.

Where the hygiene needs are met

If clients are confined to bed, either at home or in an institution, that area becomes not only their bedroom but also a dining room, living room, bathroom and toilet. It is preferable to try to reduce use of the area for multiple purposes where possible and if the client's condition permits, use of the bathroom should be encouraged. Movement and exercise are stimulating, as is a change of scenery and therefore walking or being taken to the bathroom in a wheelchair may afford time for conversation.

Some clients who can get out of bed but have limited mobility may prefer to wash by their beds and some may only require assistance with inaccessible areas such as their back or feet. Clients who are confined to bed for a short time may be able to wash in bed with minimal assistance. Finally, those clients who are too unwell to get out of bed require a bed or blanket bath (the latter so called because a blanket is used to cover the client while they are undressed and being bathed).

Skin care

The skin is a protective barrier which needs to be maintained intact. A dirty wound not matter how small could lead to a debilitating infection. The skin is the largest organ of the body and it:

- has a surface area of approximately $2\,m^2$ (two square metres)
- makes up about 15% of the total body weight
- receives stimuli perceived as pain, pressure, hot or cold
- regulates body temperature
- excretes water and salt (sweat)
- manufactures vitamin D
- screens harmful ultraviolet rays
- covers and protects inner organs.

The skin is composed of two layers: an outer epidermis of dead and dying cells and the inner dermis (true skin) which is a strong and flexible meshwork of fibres and other structures such as nerves, hair roots and oil glands. Figure 11.2 shows a section through the layers of the skin.

Skin colour

Cells called melanocytes produce the pigment melanin, which protects skin from harmful ultraviolet light. Dark-skinned people have more melanin in their skin.

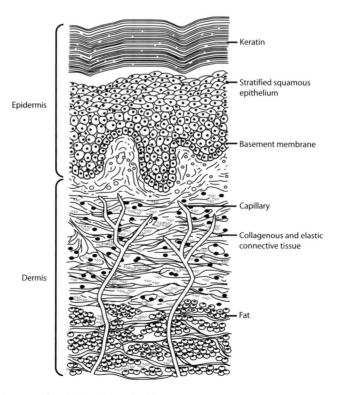

Fig. 11.2 Diagram of a section through skin.

However, melanin production reduces with age so regardless of a person's skin colour, as they age they will be more vulnerable to skin damage from exposure to sunlight[4]. Fair-skinned people are also more prone to sunburn, as well as being more at risk of skin cancer, as research studies have shown, from over-exposure to strong sunlight[5].

The skin may have small lumps or growths, moles, freckles and other discoloration of the skin – these changes being seen more with advancing age. Most are not harmful but occasionally some growths are of a serious nature such as skin cancers. Any concerns about a change to an area of skin should be reported to the registered nurse.

Dry and sensitive skin problems

Any situations or agents which reduce the water or natural oils in the skin can produce dryness and sensitivity. Dry skin is called xerosis. The following issues should be considered when providing hygiene care for clients.

Soap and detergents – prolonged or excessive use of these substances removes skin oils and causes dryness, soreness and chapping.

Perfumes – can act as irritants causing dermatitis[6], which results in intense itching with blisters and cracks.

Age – skin becomes thinner and less elastic with age, water and sebum are reduced and the skin becomes dry and wrinkled. Fragile skin is more susceptible to shearing forces so care should be taken when moving the older client[7]. Hair and nails also become brittle with age.

Hydration – a reduction in body fluid may be due to drinking less or loss of body fluids from trauma or other illness. This will have a negative effect on a client's skin and make skin damage from pressure ulcers more likely.

Skin should not be rendered too dry by excessive application of drying or irritating agents such as soaps. Skin moisture may be preserved by the use of emollients which soothe and hydrate the skin such as perfume-free creams, ointments and lotions[8]. Oils may be useful in very dry areas such as the legs or feet. However, any product that is oily or greasy may be dangerous if it causes the client to slip in the bath or on the floor. Soap substitutes and simple moisturisers can be very effective in reducing dryness. Bath cosmetics such as foams may be pleasant but can contain perfumes which irritate sensitive skin. Some clients add salt to their bath water but there is no evidence to show this provides anything but psychological benefit[9].

Some skin products can be harmful if not used appropriately. Treatments for warts may contain strong acids and skin-lightening creams can cause the skin to become friable or even permanently damaged. Some may contain harmful substances such as mercury and advice from a pharmacist or doctor should be sought before using skin products for treatments. Clients may have purchased or been given inappropriate creams and if you are unsure always check with the registered nurse.

Cosmetics

Cosmetic preparations cleanse, beautify or alter appearance and have been used by both men and women since the earliest times. However, in Western society men do not usually wear make-up in everyday life. Make-up can play an important part in maintaining body image and carers should encourage clients to maintain their normal appearance as much as possible. Some clients may use cosmetics as a camouflage to hide a blemish on the skin, for example a severe burn, scar or birthmark. However, some cosmetics that contain perfume can cause irritations.

Deodorants

Deodorants are substances which lessen offensive odours. They act by preventing the growth of the bacteria which cause that distinctive body smell. What we eat can also affect body odour, as the skin excretes the smell of some foods such as garlic. Anti-perspirants act by reducing the activity of the sweat glands in the skin, thus helping to reduce odour.

Checking for abnormalities of the skin

> **Activity 11.4**
>
> When you are washing a client you may observe some skin changes or abnormalities. From your experience of changes that can occur, make a list of abnormalities.

Your list may include:

- Rashes – may be caused by medications or contact with irritating substances. A rash may indicate a viral illness such as measles
- Inflammation or redness may be a sign that a pressure ulcer is developing
- Swelling or oedema can be due to trauma or fluid retention in the tissues caused by heart failure or renal failure (kidney failure)
- Spots or boils
- Dry flaking skin
- Bruising, cuts, burns or blisters
- Insect bites
- Changes of skin colour such as jaundice

Pruritus

Pruritus is the term used to describe itching. It can lead to scratching and skin damage. There are various causes but it is generally a response to an irritating substance such as perfume, detergents used to wash clothes, or some plants. It may be due to a medical condition or medicines such as antibiotics or infestations (see below).

Cellulitis

Cellulitis is an acute infection of the skin caused by bacteria. The skin is red, swollen, painful and the individual usually has a fever. The affected skin area may be small or a whole limb, commonly the legs[10].

Dermatitis

Dermatitis is a general term for inflammation of the skin.

Psoriasis

Psoriasis is a common non-contagious skin condition characterised by red, raised silvery scales on the skin. It can occur in different areas of the body and to different degrees. It is known to be an inherited condition[11].

Eczema

Eczema is an inflammatory condition often associated with an allergy when there is a rash with itching, blisters, and leakage of fluid from the skin or exudation.

Bathing a client

Activity 11.5

Imagine that you have become dependent on somebody else for meeting your hygiene needs. List the points you would like your carer to consider when helping you.

Your list may include some of the following:

- Privacy
- Dignity
- Consideration of any cultural customs
- Warmth
- Gentle handling
- Skill in carrying out the procedure
- Giving you an explanation before the carer acts
- Encouraging you to do things for yourself, if possible

Preparation for bathing

It is important to prevent undue exposure, and the procedure should be completed without the client becoming fatigued or cold. The care plan should detail how, when and with what level of assistance the client should be bathed.

- The procedure should be explained to the client and consent obtained.
- Pain must be relieved before commencing washing or bathing. If pain-relieving drugs are required they should be given by a registered nurse and time should then be allowed for these to take effect. This may be up to half an hour.
- Prior to washing or bathing, the client should be offered the opportunity to use the toilet.
- Furniture should be arranged so that it is not in the way. The bedside area should be clear of any obstructions. In the bathroom, there must be a chair for the client to sit down as necessary.
- Privacy should be ensured whenever the client is washed. An 'engaged' sign should be used on the bathroom door to prevent any unnecessary intrusion.
- When the client is washed in bed the height of the bed must be raised to a comfortable and safe level for the carer. This may be problematic for clients being cared for in the community and if the working height is not appropriate for the carer this must be reported as a health and safety hazard.
- In hospital or a nursing home, the client's agreement should be obtained to which toiletries and towels may be used. Clean linen will be required if the client is in bed. Suitable receptacles for dirty or soiled linen should be within easy reach, as dirty linen should not be carried about or placed on the floor.
- As with making beds it is quicker, when bed-bathing dependant clients, if you can work in pairs as the task can be completed in less than half the time.
- Collect the water in the bowl for a bed-bath only when you are ready to start otherwise it will quickly become cold. The temperature should be between 43 °C and 46 °C[12]. Do not overfill the bowl or spills may occur.

Bed-baths

Throughout this procedure, you should explain to the client what you are about to do. A blanket should cover the client, unless the room is very warm, to prevent chilling. The top bedclothes should be removed leaving the client covered by a blanket and sheet, as the bed will need remaking and linen may become damp. The top sheet is then pulled down under the blanket, which is left in place to cover the client. Then avoiding exposure of the client as much as possible, the client's nightclothes are removed.

Towels should be used to protect the bedclothes. The client is washed systematically starting, as a rule, with the face. The order of washing the limbs and trunk may depend on their specific needs. For example, if the client has been incontinent then the genital areas should be washed and the bed changed first as clients should never be left in a wet or dirty bed. The water must always be changed after cleaning the genital area. The skin should be washed with firm but gentle strokes. After applying soap or an alternative cleaning agent with a flannel or disposable cloth, the skin is rinsed and quickly dried to prevent chilling. Check that the client feels dry and comfortable.

Bathing specific areas of the body

Face and neck

Some clients may not wish to have soap on their faces and only use water. If possible, the client should wash his or her own face. If soap is used care must be taken around the eyes.

Ears

Ears should be cleansed and dried carefully.

Arms and hands

Start with the client's arm that is furthest from you. Place a towel under the arm and wash and then rinse it paying special attention to the axilla (underarm area). Dry this arm and then wash and dry the arm nearest to you. This prevents the arm that you have already washed becoming wet again. Your assistant, if you have one, can dry the first arm whilst you prepare to wash the other. Hands can be placed directly in the bowl of water which can help soften the finger nails if they require trimming.

Chest and upper abdomen

For women, the area under the breasts requires special attention. Profuse sweating may cause this area to become sore and excoriated if not kept clean and dry. Talcum powder should not be applied as it can become congealed and may increase soreness or cause fungal infection.

Upper back

If the client is able, this area can be washed with the client sitting forward if he or she is comfortable in this position. Alternatively, the client can lie on their side and the towel is then laid on the bottom sheet to prevent it becoming wet.

Buttocks and perineal area

If the client is lying on their side then the buttocks and perineal area (the area between the legs) can be washed after the upper back. The carer should wear disposable gloves and use a specially designated flannel, or preferably a disposable cloth. The water must be changed after washing this area of the body.

As the sacrum is an area where pressure ulcers are most likely to occur, especially where skin is very fragile or the client's general condition is very poor, it is essential that the cleansing is done very gently. Vigorous rubbing must be avoided, as this will tear the skin.

Legs and feet

Legs and feet are washed using the same principles as for the arms allowing the feet to be soaked in a bowl of water if necessary. Legs should be moved gently so that a towel can be placed underneath prior to washing. The calves should be observed for pain, redness and swelling as this may indicate deep vein thrombosis, a serious condition associated with immobility. The client should be encouraged if possible to move their legs and exercise their ankles on their own (active exercise). If the client is unable to move the carer may be instructed to perform passive exercises. The feet, particularly between the toes should be dried carefully. Any sign of athlete's foot, a fungal infection, which appears as an itchy, dry scaly rash between the toes, or very inflamed skin in severe cases, should be reported[13].

Genital area

If possible the client should do this part of the bath him- or herself to maintain dignity and independence. A second towel is placed between the legs to prevent the bedclothes becoming wet. As with the buttocks, a specially designated flannel or disposable cloth should be used. The carer can prepare the flannel or cloth and hand this and the towels to the client.

When washing this area for a dependent client the carer should wear disposable gloves.

When washing female clients the flannel or cloth must be wiped from front to back to prevent bacteria from the anal area contaminating the urethra, leading to urinary tract infection.

If assisting an uncircumcised male the foreskin should be drawn back to wash and dry the penis before gently replacing the foreskin. The scrotum should also be washed with care.

When washing incontinent clients special cleansing solutions may be used as an alternative to soap and water[14]. If a client particularly wishes talcum powder (talc) it must be used sparingly. Generally, talc should be avoided, especially if the skin is dry, in areas where there are folds of skin or in situations where the client is incontinent.

After the bed-bath has been completed, the client can be dressed and the bed re-made. Care should be taken to avoid pulling the client's limbs or causing friction over any bony areas as this can lead to pressure ulcers.

Disposal of linen and equipment after a bed-bath

Soiled or dirty linen should be disposed of carefully. In clients' own homes this may be dealt with immediately. In institutions personal clothing should be placed in plastic bags and labelled. It may be advisable to leave a note for the client's visitors who can remove the items quickly for laundering. Bed linen should be disposed of according to the organisation's policy. To prevent infections dirty linen must never be placed on the floor. Bowls should be washed out using the appropriate cleanser as indicated in the organisation's infection control policy. These must be dried and put away immediately and never stacked to dry in a sluice or dirty utility room as this could cause infection.

Assisted washes

If the client is able to, he or she may like to wash either in bed, sitting in a chair at the bedside with a bowl or using a basin in the bathroom, with some degree of assistance from the carer. Similar preparations should be made except that the carer may only be required to assist with certain areas such as the back or feet, depending on the client's abilities.

Bathrooms

The benefits of bathing are:

- Relaxation when tired
- Therapeutic
- Psychological (reducing stress)
- Warming

Showers

Some clients may prefer to shower. The older client may be anxious about standing but some showers have plastic seats.

Health and safety hazards in the bathroom

Specific safety measures are required in bathrooms to prevent accidents. See Chapters 7 and 8 for further details regarding health and safety.

Bath water temperature

This *must* be tested prior to the client entering the bath. In institutions, special care must be taken with hot water as it is often at a high temperature to prevent the growth of the Legionella bacteria, which thrive in warm-water systems and can cause legionnaires' disease. To prevent scalds the bath should first be filled with some cold water and then hot water added to the required temperature. The back of your hand or elbow will give a more accurate feeling of bath temperature than your fingers. Very hot baths are not recommended for clients who are ill or for clients with some skin conditions such as eczema.

Preventing falls

Non-slip surfaces should be used in baths or showers and there should be a mat for clients when they step out. Oils can make the bath more slippery as can wet floors or talcum powder on the floor. Clients in the community should be advised on how they can make their bathrooms safer.

Call buzzers

In institutions, all bathrooms and bed areas should have call bells and clients should never be left without the means to call for help. If there is any danger of a client having an epileptic fit, they should not be left alone. The registered nurse should advise on the level of supervision required.

Cleaning and preventing infection

Baths should be fully cleaned after use, and in institutions, to prevent cross-infection, the recommended cleaning agent should be used. If the client is incontinent, special care must be taken to prevent cross-infection.

Moving and handling

Bath seats and handles, transfer boards and bath hoists should be available in institutions. Adaptations can be made to the client's home and suitable hoists should be obtained if necessary. (See Chapters 7 and 8.)

Preventing exposure

When using a bath hoist, to lift a client in or out of the bath, the client's shoulders should be covered with a towel. This can help maintain dignity and warmth. Following the bath the client should be re-dressed as quickly as possible and helped to clean teeth, style hair and apply any cosmetics. After the client has left the bathroom, it should be made clean and tidy.

Mouth care

The mouth is needed to speak, eat and breathe, so if it becomes dry, dirty and diseased communication, nutrition and respiration are affected and become difficult and uncomfortable to maintain. Clients whose resistance to infection is low are more prone to developing oral infections. In fact oral diseases are the commonest form of disease in the world[15]. Mouths of dependent clients should be carefully monitored and cleaned.

The salivary glands produce about 1000 ml of saliva a day. Saliva is mostly composed of water with a substance called lysozyme, which helps to destroy harmful bacteria. Salivary production increases at the sight and smell of food. I am sure your mouth has watered at the sight or smell of your favourite dish! Another function of saliva is that it helps break down food, thus aiding digestion. As it keeps the mouth moist, it helps when chewing food (mastication) and aids swallowing. Some drugs reduce the production and flow of saliva, making the mouth unpleasantly dry, affecting eating and sometimes making speech difficult.

Clients having cancer treatments often have mouth problems. Agents used to kill cancer cells also destroy healthy cells causing inflammation and ulceration in the mouth and other parts of the digestive tract. Good mouth care can help clients' self-esteem[16].

Care of the teeth

> Every tooth in a man's head is more valuable than a diamond.
> (From 'Don Quixote' by Miguel De Cervantes 1547–1616)

When foods containing sugar and starches are eaten some of these dissolve in the saliva and are consumed by the bacteria in our mouths. A sticky mass of micro-organisms called plaque coats the teeth. The bacteria produce acids, which, if not removed by brushing, attack the enamel of the teeth causing holes or dental caries. Gums that support the teeth can also be affected by inflammation (gingivitis) and bleeding may occur when the teeth are cleaned. Gum disease can cause teeth to fall out. Losing teeth is often considered a natural part of ageing, but looking after your teeth can mean you can keep these precious items well into old age.

Preventing oral infections

If clients are taking antibiotics, they may develop an oral fungal infection, because the antibiotics that kill harmful bacteria in part of the body also destroy the normal bacteria in the mouth. This side-effect of the antibiotic means that other micro-organisms such as fungi are able to multiply in the mouth. Antifungal liquids may need to be given as treatment after the mouth has been cleaned.

Equipment for mouth care and cleaning teeth

- Toothbrush
- Toothpaste
- Mouthwash
- Sponge cleaners or swabs
- Dental floss
- White paraffin or lip salve
- Cleaning lotions

The equipment should be selected according to the client's age, ability and need. Consent should be gained from the client and the carer should wear disposable gloves when cleaning a dependent client's mouth. The care plan should be consulted to determine what assistance is required and if any specially pre-scribed solutions are required to clean the mouth. The mouth and tongue may be cleaned with special sponge cleaners or a toothbrush. However, the cleaning of a dependent client's mouth should only be undertaken by carers who have been appropriately trained to do so. Cleaning the mouth of an unconscious person should normally only be undertaken by a registered nurse.

Toothbrushes are usually the most effective means of cleaning the mouth. Older clients may need to be supervised when cleaning their mouths even if they are able to do this themselves.

If the tongue is very 'furred', it can be cleaned very gently with a soft tooth-brush. Lips may become cracked and dirty. After cleaning the lips, petroleum jelly can be applied.

Preventing dry mouths

Dry mouth may be due to dehydration, a fever, some medications or oxygen therapy. If the mouth becomes dry, the tongue furred and the lips cracked the client not only experiences discomfort but also the increased risk of oral infec-tion. Careful and regular mouth care plus adequate fluid intake, as indicated in the care plan, can prevent this discomfort. By recording how much the client has had to drink on a fluid balance chart fluid intake can be monitored. Citrus fruit juices stimulate the flow of saliva and are refreshing, especially with the addi-tion of ice in hot weather. Sucking ice cubes is another way of keeping the mouth moist. If the client is unable to eat or drink or has a very dry mouth a mouth-wash should be offered (Fig. 11.3).

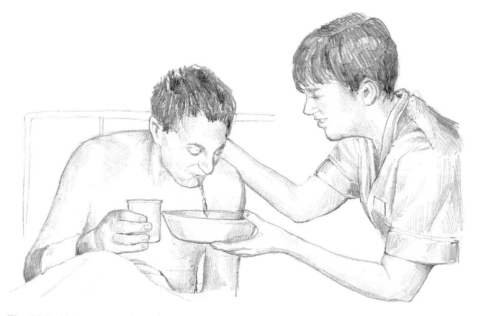

Fig. 11.3 Having a mouthwash.

Dentures

False teeth and those people who wear them are often the butt of jokes which can result in embarrassment especially when younger clients have dentures. Clients reticent about having their dentures cleaned need a sensitive approach. Dentures should be cleaned in the bathroom (never at a sink in general view of other clients or visitors or at a sink in a toilet or dirty utility area). Debris should be removed using a toothbrush or special denture brush and running water. Carers should wear disposable gloves when cleaning dentures. While the dentures are removed the mouth can be rinsed with a mouthwash and the gums gently massaged with a small soft toothbrush to keep them healthy. The dentures can be replaced in the client's mouth or placed in a denture pot in a soaking solution. Debris should be removed before soaking the denture[15]. Some clients may wish to keep their dentures in at night.

If dentures are lost, life becomes very problematic as the client cannot eat solid foods or speak clearly. Replacement of dentures can be time consuming and expensive. Dentures *must never* be wrapped in tissues as they may be mistaken for rubbish and thrown away. Dentures are valuable items and must be stored carefully in a labelled pot and kept in the vicinity of the owner.

Hair care

Hair should be brushed or combed and arranged in the client's own preferred style. This should always be done carefully as some hair types cannot tolerate vigorous brushing. For example, with clients of Afro-Caribbean origin if their hair is not combed carefully it could tear. Some hair types may require special treatments with oil or lotions to keep them in good condition.

There are approximately 100 000 hairs on the scalp and we lose about 70–100 of these each day. A hair grows about 1 mm in three days. On the scalp, this continues for about two to six years. The hair then stops growing, falls out, and a new one starts to grow in its place. Illness and certain treatments such as radiotherapy or chemotherapy (used for clients with cancer) may both increase hair loss and affect the rate of its growth.

Hair washing and drying

Activity 11.6

Think about how you feel when your hair is dirty and greasy. How does this affect your mood?

You may have identified that the situation in Activity 11.6 has a negative effect on your morale. If our hair looks dull and lifeless, this can depress our mood. Self-esteem is affected by appearance and dirty hair can have a negative effect.

Offering a client a visit to the hairdresser, an opportunity to wash their hair, or washing their hair for them can be a great morale booster.

Washing a client's hair in bed

A client's hair can be washed in the bathroom or in the bed if the client cannot get up. Explain the procedure to the client, gain consent, and collect all the equipment. The area around the bed should be cleared and the bed pulled away from the wall so that you can stand behind the bed. Remove the head of the bed and lay the client flat with their neck and shoulders well supported on pillows.

1. Explain the procedure and obtain the client's consent.
2. Protect the bedclothes by placing a plastic sheet under the client's head or use a special plastic hair-washing tray if available. This will allow dirty water to be drained away into a bucket placed on the floor at the back of the bed.
3. Collect the water and check its temperature on the inner aspects of your own wrist.
4. Using a jug, gently pour a little water over the client's head and check that it is comfortable for them. Wet the hair thoroughly before applying shampoo, and then gently massage with equal pressure from both hands to prevent shaking the head.
5. Take care to protect the client's eyes from shampoo and observe the client carefully during the entire procedure.
6. Rinse the hair with clean warm water and then towel dry.
7. Remove water and plastic sheet.
8. Replace the head of the bed then, if possible sit the client up and dry their hair with an electric hairdryer.

If the client is able, encourage them to dry and brush their own hair in their desired style. Professional hairdressers sometimes visit clients in hospital, residential homes or in their homes.

Eye care

Eyes are so precious they should always be treated with care and respect. Any abnormalities observed by carers or described by the client must be reported to the registered practitioner. If a client has discharge around their eyes, this may be an indication of infection. Following assessment, care may include taking a bacterial swab of the discharge to identify the causative organism (a registered practitioner will undertake this procedure). You may, however, be asked to carry out eye toilet to keep eyes clear.

Performing eye toilet

The procedure for eye toilet is a clean technique but packed sterile gauze swabs and normal saline solution should be used. Many units provide ready packed trays for eye toilet.

1. The procedure is explained to the client and their consent is obtained.
2. Wash and dry your hands.
3. The eye and the skin areas round it should be inspected and any features noted, e.g. swelling or redness.
4. Using a gauze swab soaked in normal saline, clean the eye by gently wiping from the inner aspect (by the nose) to the outer.
5. Use the swab once only and discard it immediately into a disposable bag.
6. Repeat the process until all the discharge is removed.
7. Take care not to contaminate the saline solution by only placing clean swabs in it.
8. Finally, use a dry swab to dry the eye and leave it comfortable.
9. Dispose of swabs and container.
10. Wash and dry your hands.

Ear care

The outer ear should be cleaned with the client's own face flannel. If there is any excessive build-up of wax (which often occurs in the older client and can affect hearing), it may need to be removed by instillation of ear drops or the ears may need to be syringed by a doctor or registered nurse.

If the client has a hearing aid this should be cleaned according to the manufacturer's instructions. Clients should be encouraged to wear their hearing aids because if they cannot hear their safety is at risk. Advice concerning battery replacement and servicing of hearing aids can be obtained from audiology departments.

Nail care

Nails are hardened skin cells which protect the fingers and toes. Fingernails grow at a rate of 1 mm a week although toe nails grow more slowly. Dirty nails can be a source of infection and therefore nails should be cleaned with the client's own nail brush or other manicure implements.

Carers should be specially trained in nail cutting before undertaking this procedure to prevent injury. Client's nails should be trimmed when necessary using appropriate equipment. Filing fingernails with a disposable emery board is preferable to cutting. Nail clippers should be used for toenails because these nails are harder and more difficult to cut especially in older people. Fingernails should be slightly rounded, while toenails should be straight to prevent them from 'in growing'.

Soaking feet in warm water prior to cutting makes the task easier but a podiatrist should see any client who has very hard or overgrown toenails. A podiatrist *must* see all diabetic clients, as the risk of infection due to skin abrasion is high.

Shaving

> Men for their sins have shaving too entailed upon their chins, a daily plague.
>
> (Byron, 'Don Juan', Canto XV1 23)

Despite the images of unshaven pop-stars, male clients who are not shaved daily appear unkempt. This can be distressing for clients and their visitors as it gives an impression of poor standards of care. Morale and self-esteem can be greatly improved by shaving.

Male carers may find this easier to begin with as they can draw on their own experiences. If you are female and have no experience of shaving men, it is advisable to try this first on a willing family member or watch carefully how it is done before shaving a client.

An electric razor is quicker and easy but only the client's razor should be used. Sharing electric razors represents an infection hazard from blood-borne microorganisms. This may be referred to as a dry shave. For wet shaves, only safety razors should be used. The blades must be sharp or cuts may easily occur. Used razors should be disposed of in the 'sharps' container. If the client has long hairs on his chin these should be clipped first as attempting to shave long hair is very painful. If the client is confined to bed, he should be supported in the upright position. If possible, the client should shave himself and in this situation all the equipment must be easily at hand. The client will need water, towels, razors, shaving foam or soap, a brush and a mirror. Normally the water for shaving should be hot but no hotter than the client can comfortably tolerate. When a client shaves himself, he may still need careful supervision, as razor blades and hot water are potentially hazardous.

If you are required to shave a client's face then follow this procedure.

1. Explain what you are going to do and gain the client's consent.
2. Moisten the area to be shaved with hot water, checking the temperature carefully, to soften the hair and skin, then apply the soap or foam.
3. Gently pull the skin taut and shave using downward strokes.
4. Avoid pressing too hard as this can cut the skin.
5. Ask the client to move his mouth in different directions to help make the skin surface taut.
6. On completion, wash away any residual soap or foam and dry the client's face.
7. Cold water or aftershave lotion may be applied at the client's request.
8. Offer the client a mirror to let him to see the result.

The client with a beard or moustache may need to have these trimmed. Prior to doing this, obtain the client's consent. However, it may be better to use the assistance of a barber if available.

Unwanted facial hair in females can be most effectively removed by using depilatory creams. If a client is dependent, it may be that she is hesitant in asking you to do this for her. However, facial hair can be a source of embarrassment for women and its removal can greatly improve self-esteem and confidence. Carers should approach this issue with sensitivity.

In some cultures, body hair can be considered unattractive and therefore hair from underarms, legs, or the pubic area is removed. Some religious groups have requirements to shave specific areas, for example some orthodox Jewish women may shave their heads and always wear wigs. Unless contraindicated on medical grounds, clients should follow their usual routines.

Hair removal prior to surgical procedures or operations

If an area where a surgical incision is to be made is excessively hairy then this may be clipped. There has been a growing trend away from shaving skin prior to surgery as it can cause skin damage and infection.

Infestations

It is easy to stand pain, but difficult to stand an itch.
(From *The importance of living*, Chang Chao 1676)

The very thought of infestation is enough to make you itch. By the time you have read this section, you may find yourself scratching imaginary insects! However, it is an important subject to consider in connection with working as a carer. Some clients requiring assistance with hygiene may be debilitated from neglect and may have become infested. Invading parasites live by sucking blood from the host after first biting the skin. The bites cause an irritant or allergic response[17]. The term 'lousy' often used nowadays to describe just feeling unwell comes from the experience of losing blood owing to infestation.

Attitudes towards clients who are infested

Peoples' attitudes to such parasites have changed. Whereas once they were accepted as a natural part of life to be tolerated, nowadays they are regarded with disgust being largely associated with vagrants, the unkempt and living in squalid conditions. This change in attitudes has accompanied the improvement in our standards of living. Clients who are infested must be treated with a caring and non-judgemental attitude on the part of the carer. Clients should be encouraged to use good personal hygiene to prevent re-infestation. The client may be homeless or have a mental health problem and the health care team will need to manage these underlying problems.

Protective clothing

When dealing with an infested client, protective clothing – disposable gloves, plastic aprons and head caps when dealing with nits, should be worn. Carers may be very worried about catching lice. However, good standards of personal hygiene and changing and laundering of uniforms or working clothes are usually adequate protection against body lice because lice are heat dependent insects and will die once away from the body.

Lice

There are three distinct types of lice, which have adapted to living on different parts of the human body. Lice feed on blood. They range in size from 2 mm to 4 mm long. Their bites cause intense itching.

Head lice (nits)

This type of lice is becoming increasingly common especially among children where close contact during play aids spread. The head louse lives in the hair on the head preferring fine, clean hair, which provides an ideal environment to lay its eggs or nits as they are commonly called. These lice are discouraged by oily conditions; therefore the child with clean hair is more likely to attract head lice, as frequent washing reduces scalp oil. Head lice lay their eggs (a female head louse can lay 10 eggs a day[18]) on hair next to the scalp, which is close to their food supply. The eggs are 1 mm long, pale cream coloured and waxy in appearance. These eggs are stuck with a glue-like substance and cannot be removed by brushing or washing with an ordinary shampoo. Nits can be removed by two methods:

- Wet combing: After washing the hair, normal conditioner (to make the hair too slippery for the lice) is applied. The hair is parted at intervals and then combed outwards from the hair root using a special fine tooth or nit comb. Nit combs can be purchased from a chemist. This needs to be repeated every three to four days over a period of two weeks.
- Washing with special insecticide shampoo or applying a lotion or oily conditioner to detach the nits.

Head lice spread very quickly in children. Parents may be embarrassed or angry to discover that their child has nits. If one child in the family has nits the rest of the family should be treated as well or re-infestation is likely to occur.

Body lice

These are much less hardy than head lice and are unable to cope with changes in body temperature. They do not live on the body surface but in the fibres and seams of clothing, only going onto the person's skin to suck blood for sustenance. Body lice live on people who wear the same clothes continuously and who do not take them off to wash.

Body lice can be treated by:

- insecticide powders and sprays
- bathing
- removal and incineration of affected clothes and bed linen.

Pubic lice or 'crabs'

These are specialised lice, which live on coarse hair, mostly in the pubic region. They have claw-like front feet to cling on to their host and only transfer to another host during sexual contact. They can be treated by special solutions. Sexual partners should be treated at the same time.

Fleas

Human fleas, which were once common, are now rare. Centuries ago men shaved their heads and wore wigs to reduce infestation. Nowadays people are more likely to be bitten by fleas from pets such as cats or dogs. If this occurs then the animal and the soft furnishings in the house should be treated. Careful vacuuming of the carpets, especially close to the walls will remove the eggs that the fleas may have laid in the carpets. Fleas and their eggs are very resilient and to kill a flea, if you catch one, you need to squash it between two hard surfaces.

Scabies

Scabies is a common infestation caused by the mite *Sarcoptes scabiei* (Greek for flesh cutter). This condition is common in children and those living in institutions, e.g. elderly care homes[19]. The mites burrow into the skin and lay eggs. When these hatch the intense itching, which is characteristic of this problem, occurs especially at night[20]. Scabies is most commonly found on the hands and under arms but can occur on other parts of the body. The rash caused by scabies may appear as fine red twisted lines. The danger is that scabies might be mistaken for other inflammations and not treated quickly. Treatment is with special lotions which should be applied according to instructions. The condition is highly contagious and carers must be careful to avoid close contact.

Bed bugs

These are not common nowadays; however, carers working in the community may occasionally encounter problems with bed bugs. The bugs live in old walls and furniture and come out at night to suck blood from humans who are asleep. If this sort of infestation occurs, the furniture may need to be fumigated or destroyed.

Summary

Effectively meeting a client's hygiene needs is the basis for good care. The client's privacy and right of choice should always be respected to ensure satisfaction with the service when providing this aspect of personal care.

References

1. Department of Health (2001) *Essence of Care – Patient-Focused Benchmarking for Health Care Practitioners*. Department of Health, London.
2. Dimond, B. (2002) *Legal Aspects of Nursing*, 3rd edition. Longman, England.
3. European Convention on Human Rights (1998) *Human Rights Act*. Articles 3 and 8. (www.echr.coe.int).
4. Penzer, R. and Finch, M. (2001) Promoting healthy skin in older people. *Nursing Standard* **15** (34), 46–52.
5. Treharne-Davies, J. (1999) Healthcare students' attitudes to sunbathing. *Nursing Standard* **13** (17), 42–45.
6. Gooch, J. (1989) Skin hygiene. *Professional Nurse* **5** (1), 13–18.
7. Smoker, A. (1999) Fungal infections. *Nursing Standard* **13** (17), 48–52.
8. Courtenay, M. (1998) Preparations for skin conditions. *Nursing Times* **94** (7), 54–55.
9. Watson, M. (1984) Salt in the bath. *Nursing Times, November Occasional Paper* **80** (19), 57–59.
10. Baxter, H. and McGregor, F. (2001) Understanding and managing cellulitis. *Nursing Standard* **15** (44), 50–52.
11. Cloote, H. (2000) Psoriasis. *Nursing Standard* **14** (45), 47–52.
12. Taylor, R. (2000) Hygiene. In Harkreader, H. (ed.) *Fundamentals of Nursing – Caring and Clinical Judgement*. W.B. Saunders Co, Philadelphia.
13. Smoker, A. (1999) Skin care in old age. *Nursing Standard* **13** (48), 47–53.
14. Whittingham, K. (1998) Cleansing regimes for continence care. *Professional Nurse* **14** (3), 167–170.
15. Jones, C.V. (1998) The importance of oral hygiene in nutritional support. *British Journal of Nursing* **7** (2), 74–83.
16. Denton, E. (1999) Mouthcare – an indicator of the level of nursing care a patient receives? *Journal of Community Nursing* **13** (11) 8, 11–12, 14.
17. Graham-Brown, R. and Bourke, J.F. (1998) *Mosby's Color Atlas and Text of Dermatology*. Mosby, London.
18. Cook, R. (1998) Treatment of head lice. *Nursing Standard* **12** (19), 49–52.
19. Hadfield-Law, L. (2001) Dealing with scabies. *Nursing Standard* **18** (31), 37–45.
20. Stewart, K.B. (2000) Combating infection. Stopping the itch of scabies and lice. *Nursing* **30** (7), 30–31.

Further reading

Buchanan, P. (1998) Dermatology. *Nursing Standard* **12** (40), 48–55.

Chapter 12

Meeting the nutritional needs of the client

Chris Flatt, Katie Cullinan and Jane Watson*

Overview

Food has a variety of roles – not only is a balanced diet essential for health, but it is also important socially and psychologically. This chapter will try to answer the following questions:

- What is a healthy diet?
- How should dietary advice differ for different client groups?
- What factors influence our client's choice of food?

Everyone has their own ideas about food and individual preferences; however, it is important not to let one's own opinions and preferences influence what your clients eat.

Key words: Healthy diet; nutritional requirements; menu planning; obesity; diabetes; heart disease; constipation; environment; food choice; eating habits; religious beliefs; vegetarianism; gastrostomy

---

Activity 12.1

Before reading any further ask yourself the question, 'Do I really eat a healthy diet?'

What is a healthy diet?

People's nutritional needs change with increasing age. Different sets of healthy eating guidelines exist for each of the following age groups:

- 0–5 years (beyond the scope of this chapter – see Further reading)
- 5 years and above
- Frail older people

*Contributer to the original version of this chapter in the first edition.

Healthy eating guidelines for the 5 years and above age group

Over the years, there have been many different messages as to what is meant by a 'healthy diet', with undue emphasis placed upon which foods are 'good' or 'bad'.

To redress the misinformation, the government issued general guidelines on healthy eating for the general public in 1991[1] (revised in 1997).

Eight guidelines for a healthy diet

(1) Enjoy your food

Healthy eating should be a pleasant experience – it doesn't mean banning some foods, but the diet should be better balanced in order to maximise health and minimise the risk of disease.

(2) Eat a variety of different foods

The wider the variety of foods eaten, the more likely it is that the diet will contain all the essential nutrients necessary for health.

(3) Eat the right amount to be a healthy weight

Being overweight leads to many health problems (see later). Eating the right diet and being physically active help to maintain correct body weight.

(4) Eat plenty of foods rich in starch and fibre

Foods such as bread, potatoes and pasta aren't themselves 'fattening'. They provide essential nutrients such as B vitamins and fibre, as well as helping to fill you up without providing too many calories. These should form a major part of everyone's diet. Most people should aim to eat more fibre – it can help protect against certain cancers and help lower blood cholesterol levels.

When dietary fibre is eaten it absorbs water and softens the stools in the gut, making them easier to pass, thus helping prevent constipation, diverticular disease and haemorrhoids. Good sources are wholemeal/high fibre cereals, wholemeal breads/pastas, fruits and vegetables.

NB: when high fibre foods are eaten it is important to drink plenty of fluid (at least 1.5 litres per day).

(5) Eat plenty of fruit and vegetables

These are essential because they provide vitamins and dietary fibre. Everyone should aim for at least five portions of fruit/vegetables every day.

(6) Don't eat too many foods that contain a lot of fat

Eating too much fat can raise cholesterol levels and increase the risk of heart disease and obesity. Most people consume too much fat and would therefore benefit from reducing their intake. There are two types of fat:

(a) saturated (found in butter, meats, dairy products, cakes, biscuits and pastries) can lead to increased cholesterol levels

(b) unsaturated (some margarines, oils, nuts and fish).

It is therefore advised to cut down the total fat intake and partially replace with unsaturated fats wherever possible.

(7) Don't have sugary foods too often

These are fine as occasional treats. However, a high intake of sugary foods in place of more nourishing foods can make the overall diet deficient in essential nutrients. Sugary foods taste good but are not filling, hence it is easy to eat excessive amounts, thereby promoting weight gain. Sweets, chocolate, desserts, sweet drinks, biscuits, cakes and sugar-coated cereals all have high sugar levels.

(8) If you drink alcohol, drink sensibly

Whilst moderate amounts of alcohol aren't harmful for most people, regularly exceeding safe drinking levels leads to progressive health deterioration, especially damage to the liver. Alcoholic drinks also contain a lot of calories and thus promote weight gain.

Recommendations used to be based on a number of 'units' of alcohol per week (1 unit=1 standard glass of wine, 1 measure of spirit, or half a pint of beer). However to discourage 'binge drinking' (where large volumes are consumed in one or two episodes, which is also very bad for one's health), the Government's Inter-Departmental Working Group on Sensible Drinking formulated new benchmarks for sensible drinking as follows[2]:

(a) Maximum daily intakes should not exceed 3–4 units per day in men and 2–3 units per day in women.
(b) Heavy sessional drinking and intoxication should be avoided.
(c) The risk of coronary heart disease in men over 40 years and post-menopausal women may be reduced by drinking 1–2 units per day.
(d) Women who are pregnant, or planning pregnancy, are advised to drink no more than 1–2 units, once or twice per week and to avoid intoxication.

Salt

On average, we eat 10 times as much salt as our body actually need every day. Half of this comes from processed foods such as crisps, salty meats, sauces and biscuits. Salt is also added to food in cooking as well as at the table. Excessive salt intake can lead to raised blood pressure, which in turn can lead to heart disease and strokes. One should try to decrease salt intake wherever possible.

Fluid

Fluid is essential to life. While humans can live without food for a period of weeks, they cannot withstand deprivation of fluid for more than a few days. In adults, water comprises 50–70% of the total body weight.

Fluid intake

This is normally regulated by the sensation of thirst, which is controlled by the brain. We obtain fluid from food as well as the drinks that we consume.

Fluid output

The kidneys mainly control fluid output, but losses also occur via the skin, lungs and gastro-intestinal tract. The level of these losses depends upon factors such as climate, activity, state of health and dietary intake.

Fluid requirements

Individual requirements for fluids vary considerably. The minimum intake should be sufficient to replace losses from all sources and provide adequate dilution for the excretion of wastes via the kidneys. A general rule is that a person requires 30–35 ml of fluid per kg body weight per day, (hence a 60 kg woman would require 1800–2100 ml per day).

Most healthy adults should aim to drink at least 1.5–2 litres per day (3–4 pints), more in hot weather or if very physically active.

Fluid balance

Long-term (or 'chronic') dehydration can lead to constipation, headaches, lethargy and mental confusion, and increased risk of urinary tract infections and kidney (renal) stones.

Activity 12.2

Compare your own diet with the established healthy eating guidelines. Do you eat a balanced diet/how could your diet be improved?

Healthy eating for frail older people

Food is essential for both physical and social well-being, whatever a person's age. However, for frail older people it is often more important to ensure that they are getting adequate nutrition rather than being over-zealous in encouraging them to follow strict healthy eating guidelines.

Fat intake

For the frail older client, fat intake should only be reduced if they are overweight. Fat is a valuable source of vitamins A and D, which are essential to maintain good health.

People often want to eat less as they become older, therefore fat can be a useful source of energy. However, as with all population groups, it is advisable not to encourage excessive amounts of fatty foods.

Sugar intake

Frail older clients should only reduce their intakes of sugar if they are trying to lose weight, have diabetes or still have their own teeth. If a client has a poor appetite, sugar can be a useful way of increasing calorie intake.

Salt intake

Older people have fewer taste buds than younger people hence cannot taste foods so well. Salt restriction should not be encouraged (unless medically indicated) as it can make food less palatable and less interesting, hence affecting the client's desire to eat.

Fibre intake

Older people are more prone to constipation, hence a high fibre diet should be encouraged. Plenty of fluids should also be encouraged, which may be more difficult in older clients who tend to have a reduced sense of thirst and may worry about incontinence, especially at night.

It is important to ensure adequate fluid intake, as constipation can itself increase urinary incontinence (a full intestine can push on the bladder).

What about vitamins and minerals?

A good supply of vitamins and minerals is essential, (see Table 12.1).

If one eats a well-balanced diet, following healthy eating guidelines, with plenty of variety and appropriate quantities then it is highly likely that we are getting enough of these. However, if one has a poor diet, or has increased requirements through illness, it may be necessary to encourage a vitamin supplement, but one should always consult with a doctor or dietitian.

Planning the menu

When planning a client's menu, there are many factors to consider. Wherever possible, the client should be encouraged to take part in this process. As a carer,

Table 12.1   Sources of important vitamins and minerals (micro-nutrients).

Vitamin	Good dietary sources	Bodily functions
Vitamin B1 (thiamin)	Wholegrain cereals, nuts, meat, fish, pulses, yeast extract	Helps in the breakdown of food to provide energy to the body
Vitamin B2 (riboflavin)	Liver, milk, eggs	As for vitamin B1
Nicotinic acid	Wholegrain cereals, meat, fish, liver, pulses	Used by the nervous system
Folic acid and vitamin B12	Liver, green vegetables, meat, eggs, yeast extract	Formation of blood; to prevent anaemia
Vitamin D	Oily fish (mackerel, herring, sardines, pilchards), eggs, margarines, breakfast cereals	Helps to keep bones healthy
Calcium	Cheese, milk, yoghurt, fish, pulses	Helps keep bones and teeth healthy (with vitamin D)
Vitamin C	Citrus fruits and their juices, squashes, green vegetables and potatoes	Helps the absorption of iron; helps body fight infections (an 'antioxidant')
Iron	Liver, kidney, red meats, wholemeal bread, dried fruit	Formation of blood

you can help, encourage, advise and support your clients in this process, but they must have the final say in choosing the foods that they eat.

When planning a menu try to ensure that:

- The client's individual food preferences have been taken into account
- The nutritional recommendations have been met (Table 12.2)
- Any special dietary needs have been taken into account (such as diabetes)
- A wide variety of foods and cooking methods have been used
- A sufficient variety of colour, texture and taste have been included in the meals
- The meal is within the budget of the client or catering department
- The meal is served at the appropriate time for the client
- The cooking practices follow the current Food Hygiene Regulations

It is essential that a client's own food preferences and needs are recognised and respected.

Daily nutritional targets

These can be used to help plan a client's menu. It must be stressed that these are only **guidelines** for the minimum amounts needed each day; the actual amounts will vary according to age, sex and activity levels (Table 12.2).

Monitoring food and drink intake

It may be necessary to monitor a client's food and drink intake in order to ensure that they are eating the correct quantity and type of food, and/or taking sufficient amounts of fluid.

Table 12.2   Daily nutritional targets.

Food	Quantity	Comments
Milk	$1/4$–$1/2$ litre ($1/2$–1 pint) per day	Cheese/yoghurt/bony fish are also good sources of calcium
	Two portions from this list daily:	–
Meat	60–90 g cooked weight	
Fish	120–150 g cooked weight	
Cheese	60 g	
Eggs	1 large/2 small	
Pulses (beans/peas)	60 g dried weight	
Bread	At least one portion from the list at each meal	Use wholemeal/whole-wheat varieties/brown rice to increase fibre content
Breakfast cereal		
Pasta		
Rice		
Potatoes		
Vegetables (fresh or frozen) and salad	At least 2 portions per day	
Fruit (fresh, stewed, tinned or dried or	At least 2–3 portions per day	
Fluid	At least 8 cups of fluid per day	

Monitoring usually takes the form of Food Record Charts (FRC) – the quantity and type of food eaten should be recorded as accurately as possible. For example, if a sandwich is eaten, one should record how many slices of bread, whether white or wholemeal, the sandwich filling and how much of it was actually eaten. The more accurate the data collected, the more useful it will be.

If a client is obviously not meeting their daily food or drink requirements, it is important to notify the appropriate member of the health care team as soon as possible.

Activity 12.3

Complete your own food and drink chart for one whole day, accurately recording the quantities taken. Compare this to the nutritional targets given earlier to see whether or not you are having the correct amount of food and drink.

Swallowing and swallowing difficulties

Normal swallowing process

When you eat and drink you do so without thinking. If something goes wrong you soon realise how important it is to have your face and mouth in full working order so you can eat and drink comfortably. (Think what it is like when you have an anaesthetic injection at the dentist and you dribble when you drink.)

For normal swallowing to take place muscles in your cheeks, lips, tongue, soft palate, throat and those going down to the stomach need to work properly. Normal swallowing can be divided into three main stages (Fig. 12.1) involving:

- The mouth (oral stage)
- The throat (pharyngeal stage)
- The oesophagus (the muscular tube from the throat to the stomach, thus the oesophageal stage)

Oral stage (Fig. 12.1a,b)

This is the only part of swallowing of which you are consciously aware, but where does it begin? Some people think that it begins before any food or drink passes your lips. This is supported by clinical experience which shows that the more one can do to help a person to get ready to eat or drink and to feed themselves, the more normal the whole swallowing process.

Factors that influence this pre-oral stage include hunger, thirst, smell and appearance of the food, oral hygiene, physical ability, posture, surroundings and emotional considerations such as stress and mood.

Once you take a bite of food you chew it and move it around in your mouth, mixing it with saliva until it is soft enough to swallow. With your tongue and cheeks you make the food into a ball (bolus) in the middle of your mouth for

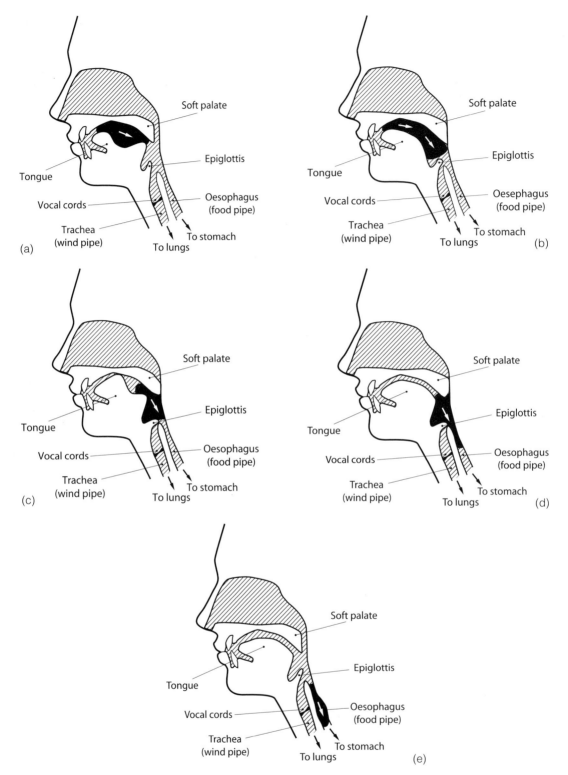

Fig.12.1 (a,b) The oral stage. (a) The food or drink is positioned for swallowing. (b) The food or drink is pushed to the back of the mouth and the swallowing reflex triggered. (c,d) The pharyngeal stage. The food or drink passes down the back of the throat. (e) The oesophageal stage. The food or drink carries down on its way to the stomach.

very small amounts of food or towards the back of your mouth for larger amounts of soft food and hard food. It is then pushed to the back of your mouth with your tongue before the reflex part of swallowing begins. It is similar with a sip of drink, only you don't chew it but form a bolus straight away in the middle of your mouth.

Pharyngeal stage

Once the swallowing reflex is triggered everything is automatic and you cannot interrupt the process. The soft palate at the back of your mouth lifts up and back so that food or drink cannot get up your nose as the bolus is squeezed into your throat. At the same time your voice box (larynx) closes, lifts up and tilts forward to make way for the bolus and you stop breathing momentarily while the food or drink is squeezed further down your throat (Fig. 12.1c). The epiglottis folds down over the entrance to the wind pipe (trachea) to stop the food or liquid going down the wrong way into your lungs (Fig. 12.1d). Once the bolus enters the oesophagus, the larynx returns to its normal position and breathing resumes.

Oesophageal stage

The bolus is squeezed the whole length of the oesophagus by its muscular walls contracting in waves (peristalsis) until it reaches the stomach (Fig. 12.1e). Swallowing is now finished and digestion begins.

Activity 12.4

Put your first, second and third fingers over your voice box. Swallow. Feel your voice box move up and down as you start and finish the swallow.

What causes swallowing difficulties?

Swallowing difficulties (dysphagia) can be caused by a variety of disorders ranging from stroke, Parkinson's disease, multiple sclerosis and head injury to laryngectomy (removal of the voice box).

What happens in dysphagia?

In the mouth

You may notice that the person you are caring for is drooling or having difficulty chewing or moving food around the mouth. They may not be able to clear food from the sides of the mouth. This is often due to poor control of the lips, tongue and cheeks and poor sensation in the mouth. Other problems you may notice during this stage are loss of taste and smell.

In the throat

The person you are caring for may cough or choke when eating or drinking. This might be because the swallowing reflex is delayed or absent (e.g. after a stroke) so the food or drink is either incompletely swallowed or trickles down the back of the throat into the wind pipe (trachea). Because the automatic part of swallowing has not started or is incomplete, the epiglottis has not folded down and the vocal cords are not shut. This process of food or liquid going down the wrong way and entering the wind pipe is called aspiration. It is potentially very dangerous as the lungs are designed for air, so if food or drink get in, a chest infection is likely to develop and may cause breathing complications such as pneumonia.

In the oesophagus

It is difficult to observe problems during this stage, but a person may complain of discomfort in their chest soon after they swallow.

Care required for adults with swallowing difficulties

When you are with someone who has swallowing difficulties you can help in a number of ways.

Observation

- What helps the person to swallow? For example, soft food, cold food, smooth, thick drinks.
- Which foods does the person find more difficult to swallow?

Posture

- Observe how a person is sitting, check with the illustration on the next page. Posture should be as upright as possible so that food is helped by gravity to go down the right way (Figs 12.2 and 12.3).

Consistency of food and drink

- Think about the different textures and consistencies of food (e.g. soft food may be easier to swallow than hard food which requires a lot of chewing). If clients require food of a specific consistency, make their diet as interesting as possible and try to use a variety of different foods. Try to ensure that your clients are meeting their daily nutritional targets.
- When helping someone to eat, give only one consistency at a time in small amounts.
- Look to see which liquids are easier to swallow (e.g. thick, smooth soup rather than tea).

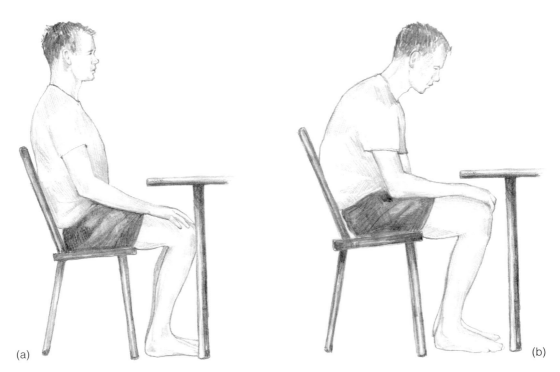

Fig.12.2   Posture: (a) good position at table and (b) bad position at table.

- Look to see if it is easier to sip from a cup or suck through a straw.
- Contact your local speech and language therapist or dietitian for further information on a specific client's individual needs.

Timing

- Allow plenty of time when someone is eating. Let your client dictate the pace, while encouraging and assisting them to self-feed as much as possible.

Temperature

- In general, cold liquids and food are easier to swallow than hot.

Remember that being fed is rarely a pleasant experience, so try to make it as agreeable as possible by doing things the way your client wishes. Sit down, try not to rush the client, and don't try to make conversation – it is impossible to chew, swallow and speak at the same time. Always ask advice from members of the team involved in the care of someone with swallowing difficulties before helping them to eat or drink. In particular consult the speech and language therapist, the dietitian and the physiotherapist.

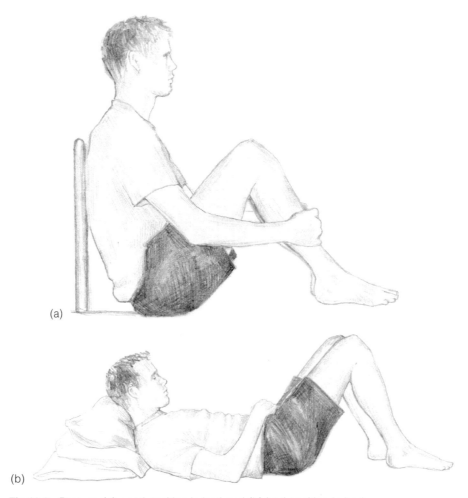

(a)

(b)

Fig.12.3 Posture: (a) good position in bed and (b) bad position in bed.

Activity 12.5

Get a dry biscuit and a cup of water. Take a bite of biscuit – bend your head to the side – now try to swallow. Have a sip of water – try to swallow with your mouth wide open. Give someone else something to eat or drink. Ask someone to feed you. How does it feel?

How to deal with a choking emergency

Be calm and reassuring.

Try to remove any visible obstruction. STOP if there is any risk of pushing the obstruction further down from the back of the mouth. Try to get the person to cough up the obstruction by hitting them firmly between the shoulder blades with the heel of your hand. Do this up to five times. If this does not work, encourage the person to lean forward with their head lower than their chest. Repeat the firm hits between the shoulder blades. If this does not work, call for help.

Therapeutic diets

This section will look at some common therapeutic diets. If you would like more detailed advice on these or other special diets, or are worried about a particular client, then please contact your local dietitian.

Obesity and the weight-reducing diet

Obesity is a very common and increasing nutritional problem. It can lead to disorders such as high blood pressure, diabetes, gall stones, stroke and coronary heart disease. Obesity occurs when a person consistently consumes more calories than their body requires. This extra energy is then stored as body fat.

The principle of a weight-reducing diet is to take in less energy than the body needs so that the body fat stores are used up. However, it is still important to have a good daily intake of all essential nutrients.

Clients needing to lose weight for medical reasons should receive individual dietary advice by a state registered dietitian.

For general weight reduction, the following guidelines are used:

- Encourage three meals every day.
- Between-meal snacks (other than fruit) should be avoided.
- Sweet and fatty foods (sweets, cakes and biscuits) should be avoided.
- Low calorie/sugar-free drinks, artificial sweeteners are beneficial, but 'diabetic' foods and slimming aids should be avoided.
- Fresh fruit or very low fat yoghurts should be encouraged in place of other puddings.
- Weight loss should be at a slow, steady rate, $\frac{1}{2}$–1 kg (1–2 lb) per week is ideal.
- Activity should be increased wherever possible, taking the individual's own ability into consideration.

If a person is very overweight, it will take many months before a target weight is achieved. During that time, plenty of encouragement and support should be provided.

Weight loss for older people is often particularly difficult as they are often unable to exercise and need only relatively small amounts of food each day (as energy requirements generally decrease with age). Before it is suggested that an elderly person follow a weight reducing diet it is important to establish who will benefit – the carers or the client? If it is not the client, then they should not be encouraged to follow a strict diet which will affect their quality of life considerably and may then lead to malnutrition.

> **Activity 12.6**
>
> If you needed to lose weight, list the changes that you could make to your diet in order to promote weight loss at a steady rate. If you lost 1 kg (2 1b) per week, how long would it take to reach your target weight?

Diabetes

Diabetes is a disorder in which the body is unable to adequately control the amount of sugar (glucose) in the blood, which is essential if the body is to function properly.

What happens normally?

Sugar is absorbed from the gut into the bloodstream. The pancreas (a gland in the abdomen) produces a hormone called *insulin*, which allows the sugar to pass into the tissues of the body where it can be used as energy.

What happens when a person has diabetes?

In diabetes the pancreas is unable to produce enough insulin to allow the sugar to move from the blood into the tissues. The sugar is therefore 'trapped' in the blood and, unless treated, sugar levels will rise uncontrollably.

When the blood sugar level is too high, small amounts of sugar over-flow into the urine, which can lead to several problems:

- Sugar draws water into the urine, making the diabetic person want to urinate frequently throughout the day and night.
- As this extra water is lost, the body becomes dehydrated, causing extreme thirst.
- Sugar in the urine is an excellent breeding ground for bacteria and can lead to urinary tract infections.

There are more serious long-term side effects of diabetes (such as damage to the nerves, kidneys, eyes and feet). The likelihood of getting these increases if the client does not follow the correct treatment for their diabetes.

Treatment

There are three main types of treatment for diabetes:

- Diet alone
- Diet and oral tablets
- Diet and insulin injections

Whatever treatment is taken, the client should always be encouraged to follow a healthy diet. There is no special 'diabetic diet', clients should simply be encouraged to follow the general healthy eating recommendations as discussed earlier in this chapter. It is important that diabetic control is monitored regularly and reviewed by the appropriate health care team as treatment often changes with increasing age.

Specific dietary points that are applicable are as follows:

- Eat regular meals containing **fibre-rich** starchy foods (bread, rice, potato and cereal).
- **Do not** miss meals.
- It may be necessary to take **between-meal snacks** to prevent the risk of low blood sugar levels (hypoglycaemia).
- **Avoid** excessively sweet/sugary food and drink, especially between meals.
- **Avoid** diabetic products – they are expensive, not low calorie and may contain a sweetener (sorbitol) which in excess can lead to diarrhoea. Diabetic/low sugar jams and squashes **should**, however, be encouraged.
- **Avoid** being overweight (can worsen blood sugar control).
- Alcohol may be taken, but not on an empty stomach. Sweet alcoholic drinks should be **avoided**.

This is only general advice and you may find that specific, individual advice may vary slightly.

Hypoglycaemia

Diabetic clients taking insulin or certain tablets may be at risk of hypoglycaemia, (a 'hypo'). This is when the blood sugar level falls to dangerously low levels and may occur when:

- A person misses a meal or snack
- Not enough starchy food is eaten
- Strenuous exercise over and above usual levels is undertaken
- More insulin (or tablets) is taken than is needed
- Excessive alcohol is consumed

Early warning signs vary from person to person, but include trembling, confusion, sweating, tingling sensations, palpitations and becoming absent-minded or argumentative. Diabetic clients usually recognise their own symptoms and thus should know when to take suitable treatment.

Hypoglycaemia should **always be treated immediately** otherwise the client may lose consciousness and ultimately could suffer brain damage or even die.

How should one treat hypoglycaemia?

If a client exhibits the above symptoms, try to get them to take one of the following:

- 50 ml Lucozade
- 3 Dextrosol tablets/boiled sweets
- Two lumps/teaspoons sugar

- Small cupful of ordinary coke/lemonade (not 'diet' types) or fresh orange juice
- 25 ml undiluted Ribena

This should make them feel better within a few minutes; however it is then important to ensure that they have a starchy snack as soon as possible, such as:

- A cup of milk and a biscuit
- A slice of toast or a sandwich
- Two digestive-type biscuits
- a bowl of cereal
- or if it is time for their next meal then this should include a normal sized portion of bread/potatoes/rice/pasta

If your client has frequent episodes of hypoglycaemia, their doctor should be informed as soon as possible.

What if your client with diabetes becomes ill?

If a client taking insulin or diabetic tablets becomes ill, it is very important that they continue taking their medication. This is because illness (even colds, influenza, diarrhoea) will cause a natural rise in blood sugar level. Non-diabetic people can cope with this, but diabetic people must continue their medications in order to help control it. It is also important for the client to continue to eat regular meals. If they do not have a good appetite, at least encourage frequent snacks throughout the day such as bread and soup, milky drinks, yoghurts and sandwiches.

Weight loss and poor appetite

Weight loss occurs when a client's dietary intake is poor or when illness causes an increased energy requirement, i.e. more energy is being used than consumed.

Nutritional intake can be increased by encouraging small, frequent meals and snacks regularly throughout the day and by offering foods which are enjoyed/attractively presented. Avoid giving large portions, as this can be very off-putting for someone with a reduced appetite.

Foods containing a high nutritional value (high protein/energy content) should be encouraged. Try offering milky drinks in place of tea/coffee/squash. Milk itself can be fortified by adding two to three tablespoons of skimmed milk powder to a pint (0.47 litre) of normal milk and then using this in tea/coffee/cereals/puddings. Extra fat and or sugar can be added to meals to increase energy intake ('food fortification').

Dietary supplements are a useful way of adding extra nourishment to the diet. These are products that contain a relatively high concentration of nutrients in a small volume. Dietary supplement can be bought in chemists, health-food shops and supermarkets (Build-Up/Complan) or are prescribable items (Fortisip, Ensure Plus, Enlive, Fresubin).

Food fortification and/or supplementation should be under the care of a dietitian. Reduced body weight is only one indicator of a poor diet – overweight clients can also become malnourished. Deficiencies of other nutrients can occur while body weight remains constant – skin changes, poor wound healing, anaemia and mood changes may all be indicators of nutrient deficiency. If you feel that your client is at risk of or has nutritional deficiencies, you should notify the health care professionals as soon as possible.

Eating for a healthy heart

The general healthy eating guidelines previously described form the basic dietary information. Two especially important factors in heart disease are obesity (if overweight then encourage weight loss) and the fat content of the diet. Broadly speaking, there are two types of fat in the blood – cholesterol and triglycerides. Raised levels of either type in the blood can increase the risk of heart disease.

General advice if a client has raised blood fat levels:

- **Total fat** intake should provide no more than 35% of the total daily energy intake, so if the daily consumption is 2000 calories no more than 70–75 g should be fat.
- The proportion of **unsaturated fats** should be relatively increased – by substituting the reduction in saturated fats with smaller amounts of polyunsaturated and monounsaturated fats (vegetable/olive oils and oily fish).
- Excessive intake of **cholesterol-rich foods** should be avoided (liver, kidney, egg yolks and shellfish).
- **Dietary fibre** can help to reduce cholesterol levels and thus fibre-rich foods should be encouraged wherever possible.
- Clients should also be encouraged to restrict both their **alcohol** and **refined carbohydrate** (sugar) intakes, as both are sources of excessive low nutritional value calories, and can increase triglyceride levels.

Factors affecting food choice

There are many factors that influence our choice of foods.

Religious beliefs

Most religions have rules or conventions about food, used as expressions of orthodoxy and unity between members of a faith. It is important to clarify an individual client's dietary requirements. Some general rules are discussed below.

Hinduism

- Most Hindus don't eat meat or fish but some may eat lamb, chicken or white fish.

- Strict Hindus may not eat eggs since they are potentially a source of life.
- Animal fats such as dripping, lard and some margarines are not acceptable. Replacements include ghee (clarified butter) and vegetable oils.
- Strict Hindus are unwilling to eat food if the utensils used in the preparation/serving of food have come in contact with meat or fish.
- Some Hindus fast for one or two days a week and this may involve missing one or more meals each day, or abstinence from everything except dairy produce or fruit and nuts all day.

Islam

- Pork and all products of pigs or certain carnivorous animals are forbidden.
- All meat should be ritually slaughtered (halal); kosher meat may be acceptable.
- Alcohol, including that used in cooking, is forbidden.
- All healthy adult Muslims must fast for the first 30 days of Ramadan – they are not permitted to eat or drink between dawn and dusk.

Sikhism

- Some, especially women, are vegetarian but they may eat chicken, lamb and fish.
- They are unlikely to eat beef or pork.

Judaism

- Pork and all products of pigs are forbidden.
- Fish with scales and fins are allowed; shellfish are not.
- Meat and milk must not be served at the same meal or cooked together.
- All meat and poultry must be kosher, i.e. must undergo a ritual method of slaughter.

Rastafarianism

- Pork and all vine products – currants, raisins, grapes and wine are forbidden.
- Most Rastafarians are vegan or vegetarian, some will eat fish.
- Processed foods/additives are avoided as much as possible.
- Frozen food is acceptable, but canned or tinned foods are not.
- Wholemeal foods are considered beneficial and are preferred to refined products.
- Alcohol is not permitted.

Cultural influences

Traditional foods vary from one culture to another and have evolved over many years, largely based on the plants most suitable for growth in that particular region (potatoes in Ireland or rice in Asia/Africa for example) and on the wildlife or domesticated animals available.

In recent years, foods have become widely available from all areas of the world, so it is unnecessary for people from other countries and cultures living in Britain to change to traditional British foods. Every effort should be made to cater for individual cultural differences wherever possible.

Personal ethics/beliefs – vegetarian and vegan diets

Vegetarians do not eat meat or poultry and some extend this to not eating fish, eggs or dairy products. The degree of exclusion is based upon the individual's religious or moral beliefs. Vegans do not eat any animal products at all.

Since meat and other animal products are valuable sources of protein in the diet, other sources of protein such as pulses (beans, peas and lentils) and their products (such as soya milk and tofu) must be included in order to prevent nutritional deficiencies from occurring.

Vegetarian diets can be a healthy way of eating if they are well planned. If unsure, there are lots of books available, or request more specific information from a dietitian.

Other factors affecting food choice

There are many physical, psychological and environmental factors that affect food choice.

Poor dentition/chewing difficulties

The ability to chew food is reduced if clients have tooth decay, poorly fitting dentures, sore/infected gums, mouth ulcers or no teeth at all. Encourage appropriate dental treatment as necessary.

Dysphagia (difficulty swallowing)

See section on swallowing.

Taste and smell

If the taste or smell of food changes, as a result of strokes, drug treatments, radiotherapy and ageing, foods which were once appealing can seem bland, tasteless or even sour or metallic. Adding pepper, vinegar, mustard, herbs, spices and dressings can improve acceptability.

Communication difficulties

Good communication is essential if clients are to make their own, informed choices of food and drink. Referral to a speech and language therapist should be encouraged if communication is poor.

Poor vision

Well-presented, attractive food can influence food choice. Eating and drinking aids may be useful.

Breathing difficulties

In order to swallow, it is necessary to stop breathing momentarily. People who have breathing difficulties can therefore find it difficult to eat much at any one time.

Offer small regular meals/drinks of high nutritional value.

Constipation and incontinence

Constipation causes feelings of fullness, nausea, general distress and decreased appetite. Encourage high fibre foods with plenty to drink.

Fear of urinary incontinence often leads to clients avoiding regular fluid intake – this can cause constipation, which worsens urinary incontinence (a full bowel presses on the bladder). Encourage to drink more during the day and less late at night.

Drugs

Many drugs have side-effects which can interfere with food intake by affecting appetite, causing nausea, diarrhoea or constipation and even reduce the ability of the body to absorb certain nutrients. If you notice any such side-effects, refer to your health care team.

Mental health problems

Dementia, confusion, depression and anxiety can all result in a change in nutritional intake. Communicating with the client can become poor and they may not express their food preferences or needs.

Some mental health problems can lead to hyperactivity, which will lead to increased nutritional requirements.

Environmental/social factors

Food choice availability, the way a meal is served and the environment a client is expected to eat in all affect the nutritional intake. Factors to consider are:

- Serving food at a client's preferred times
- Allowing clients to eat at their own pace
- Making mealtimes a highlight of the day (Fig. 12.4)
- Encouraging freedom to choose where to sit/with whom
- Removing distractions/turning off televisions

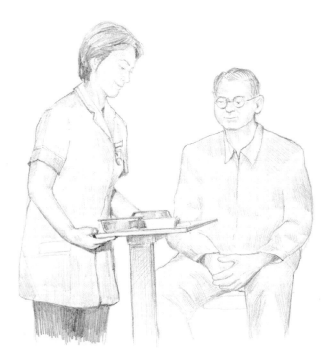

Fig.12.4 Lunch is served.

Gastrostomy feeding

A gastrostomy tube is a means of providing supplementary food and/or fluid directly into the stomach. They are used for clients who are unable to take any food or drink safely via mouth, or cannot consistently take sufficient amounts to ensure that they meet their daily requirements. An individual feeding regimen is designed depending on the desired goals of nutritional support for that specific client.

Any concerns should be discussed with the appropriate health care professional (usually a dietitian).

Summary

- An adequate and appropriate intake of food and drink is essential for good health.
- Be familiar with normal eating habits, and be aware of any consistent changes.
- Always discuss concerns with the health care team.
- Obtain the agreement of the health care team before making any changes to your client's diet.
- Be aware of any factors affecting the client's intake – therapeutic diets, religious beliefs, swallowing problems, etc.

- Mealtimes should be an enjoyable occasion – ensure that the environment is conducive to eating and that food is attractively presented.
- As a carer, you can help, support and encourage your client to eat a balanced, healthy diet, but ultimately you must respect their wishes.

References

1. Department of Health (1991) *Dietary Reference Values for Food Energy and Nutrients for the United Kingdom.* (Report on Health and Social Subjects, 41). HMSO, London.
2. Department of Health (1995). *Sensible Drinking: Report of an Inter-Departmental Working Group.* HMSO, London.

Further reading

Department of Health (1992) *The Nutrition of Elderly People* (Report on Health and Social Subjects, 43). HMSO, London.

Foodsense (1992) *The Food Safety Act 1990 and You. A Guide for the Industry.* HMSO Publication PB0 351. Available from Foodsense, London.

Garrow, J.S.J. and Ralph, W.P.T. (2000) *Human Nutrition and Dietetics*, 10th edition. Churchill Livingstone, London.

Health Education Authority (1990) *Guide to Healthy Eating.* Available from health promotion departments.

Health Education Authority (1990) *From Milk to Mixed Feeding.* Available from health promotion departments.

Langley, J. (1998) *Working with Swallowing Disorders.* Speechmark/Winslow Press, Bicester.

Longemann, J.A. (1998) *Evaluation and Treatment of Swallowing Disorders.* Pro-Ed, Austin, Texas.

Marks, L. and Rainbow, D. (2001) *Working with Dysphagia.* Speechmark/Winslow Press, Bicester.

O'Loughlin, G. and Shanley, C. (1996) *Swallowing . . . on a Plate: A Training Package for Nursing Home Staff Caring for Residents with Swallowing Problems.* Centre for Education and Research on Ageing, Concord.

O'Loughlin, G. and Shanley, C. (1998) Swallowing Management in the Nursing Home: A Novel Training Response. *Dysphagia* **13**, 172–183.

Thomas, B. (2001) *Manual of Dietetic Practice*, 3rd edition. Blackwell Science, Oxford.

Williams, K. (1991) *Practical Approach to Caring.* Pitmans, London.

Useful addresses

Department for Environment, Food and Rural Affairs, London SW1P 3J, 0207 238 6000.
Food Standards Agency, London WC2B 6NH 0207276 8000 (now incorporating MAFF).

Chapter 13

Promoting comfort, rest and sleep and caring for the client in pain

Patricia Cronin, Judith Trendall, Karen Gillett, Christine McMahon*
and Elizabeth Atchison*

Overview

This chapter has three sections. The first section covers the overall comfort of the client and discusses how we can prevent pressure ulcers (decubitus ulcers) and the complications of immobility. Bed making, positioning the clients and the use of aids to prevent pressure ulcers are included.

In the second section, an explanation of the circadian rhythm and the stages of sleep is given along with how we can promote sleep and adapt the environment and routine to facilitate sleep and rest.

Pain and its transmission are explored in the last section along with how to recognise when a client is in pain. The use of pain-killing drugs (analgesics) and the factors that affect the expression of pain are discussed. The final topic of discussion is how we as carers can help clients who are in discomfort or pain.

Key words: Immobile; pressure area; decubitus ulcer; hyperaemic reaction; necrosis; shearing; contractures; deep vein thrombosis; exercise active/passive; position; circadian rhythm; stages of sleep; routines/behaviours; insomnia; environment; nursing intervention; acute/chronic pain; analgesia; pain threshold; pain pathway

Pressure ulcers

I am sure that you have sat on a hard chair for a long time and been left feeling numb and sore. You will have consciously registered this discomfort and if the situation allowed it you would have wriggled in your seat or got up and walked about. The same also happens at night when you are asleep where you unconsciously change your position many times.

*Contributer to the original version of this chapter in the first edition.

Activity 13.1

Can you list reasons that could prevent a person changing their position when they become uncomfortable, providing they were aware of their discomfort.

Your list may include:

- Someone who is very weak and unable to move, especially if the bed clothes are restrictive
- A person who has had a stroke and lost the use of one or more parts of their body
- A person with a fractured limb (e.g. leg) who is in traction or plaster
- A person who has recently had major surgery and who may have pain or has wound drains or intravenous infusions in place
- A person whose weight does not allow them to move with ease

Sometimes a person may not be aware of their discomfort – examples include:

- A deeply unconscious person
- A person in the process of having surgery and who is lying on a hard operating table

In the case of a person who is unable to change position without assistance, the skin is subject to pressure. Areas of skin particularly prone to this are those covering a bone on which we sit or lie. The supply of blood is reduced and after a period of time the tissues in the area will be affected by the lack of oxygen and nutrients normally transported by the blood to feed the body's cells. The length of time this takes to happen varies between individuals but it is important to note that it can happen in a very short period of time particularly in vulnerable people (see below). The cells die (necrosis) and a breakdown of the skin will result in a pressure ulcer (decubitus ulcer). The destruction of the tissues is more extensive close to the bone and what you see on the skin surface does not give a clear indication of the true extent of the tissue damage.

Factors that increase the risk of developing a pressure ulcer

Factors that increase the risk of developing a pressure ulcer are generally grouped into two categories:

- External
- Internal

External factors

These include pressure, shear and friction. Pressure is the most important factor in the development of pressure ulcers and occurs when the soft tissue of the body is compressed between a bony prominence and a hard surface.

Shear occurs when the soft tissues and the skeleton move but the skin does not. This most typically happens when a client slides down the bed. According to Dealey[1] one of the main culprits of shearing is the back-rest of a hospital bed, which encourages sliding. However, it is important to note that shear can also result from sitting in an unsuitable chair. If the chair does not provide sufficient support, gravity may cause the person to slide[2]. As a result the capillaries in the skin are stretched and damaged and the blood supply to the tissues is interrupted.

Friction occurs when two surfaces rub together. Although many health care settings have or are working towards a 'no lifting policy' when moving clients, friction most commonly occurs when a person is 'dragged' across or up the bed. This causes the top layer of the skin to be scraped off.

Activity 13.2

Place your lower arm on a table with the elbow at the edge. Pressing down hard on your arm, pull your elbow towards you and over the end of the table.
   You will note that your skin stays in the same place whilst your bones (radius and ulna) move. This is shearing.

Internal factors

There are multiple internal factors that impact on the development of pressure ulcers. These can be classified under the following headings:

- Physical
- Medical/surgical
- Psychological
- Lifestyle
- Unchangeable

Physical factors

General health: Although it is not clear why, the body appears to be able to withstand greater pressure when the person is generally healthy than when ill.

Poor nutrition: People who have a poor diet lacking in carbohydrate, iron, vitamin C, proteins and minerals such as zinc are more prone to developing pressure ulcers[3]. These are needed to formulate haemoglobin in the red blood cells to aid transport of oxygen to the body's cells for energy and to keep skin generally healthy. A reduced nutritional status affects the elasticity of the skin. Skin that is dry perhaps because of a poor or reduced fluid intake is also more susceptible to damage from pressure.

Mobility: As previously mentioned, being unable to move independently is a very important factor in the development of pressure ulcers. It is important to remember that a pressure ulcer can occur whenever a person is immobile whether or not they are in bed. Tight clothing especially jeans or buttons on seat pockets can cause pressure leading to a pressure ulcer.

Skin condition: Not everybody's skin is the same and people who have paper thin skin, very dry skin, previously damaged skin or those with swelling (oedema) are more susceptible to pressure damage.

Restlessness: People who are agitated, confused, in pain or generally restless have an increased risk of developing pressure ulcers.

Medical/surgical factors

Cardiovascular system: The cardiovascular system needs to be strong to circulate the blood around the body. A poor blood supply causes malnutrition in the tissues and increases the risk of developing pressure ulcers. Conditions that affect the body's ability to circulate the blood around the body include heart disease, diabetes or surgery. In addition, some conditions such as anaemia affect the quality of the blood being circulated.

Continence: Incontinence of urine or faeces can cause maceration (softening and break up) of the skin and so increase the risk of pressure ulcers. A client who is incontinent may also be subjected to constant washing, which removes the body's natural oils thus drying the skin[4].

Medications: Medications can cause an increased risk of developing pressure ulcers. Examples include some antibiotics, steroids and sedatives.

Surgery: As mentioned earlier surgery can affect the person's ability to mobilise either through the presence of pain, drains or infusions. During surgery, a person can be immobile on the operating table for a long period of time although operating theatres now have pressure-relieving devices for use in these cases.

Psychological factors

Emotional stress: If a person is experiencing emotional stress it may affect sleep or the motivation to move themselves about or take active steps to prevent pressure ulcers.

Lifestyle factors

Smoking: People who smoke often develop narrowing of the arteries and have a reduced respiratory function (breathing). Both of these can affect the amount of oxygenated blood getting to the tissues and so increase the risk of developing pressure ulcers.

Weight/build: If a person is underweight there is less tissue covering the bones and therefore less cushioning. This causes increased pressure on the tissues. On the other hand, people who are overweight have increased pressure on the areas of the body where the amount of tissue covering the bone is thin, for example the heels or sacrum of a person who is in bed. In addition, sweat may be trapped between rolls of fat causing maceration of the skin. People who are very overweight may also find it more difficult to move particularly if one of the other factors is present, like surgery or pain.

Unchangeable factors

Age: Although pressure damage can occur in children and babies, the older person is more likely to suffer pressure damage. As people become older, their skin becomes thinner and less elastic. Older people also tend to have some wasting and are more likely to have chronic illnesses or diseases that may affect development of pressure ulcers. It is also harder for a pressure ulcer to heal in an older person than in a younger one.

Visual indicators of pressure ulcer development

Activity 13.3

Place one arm on a table and then lean your other elbow on it and press down. How does it feel? Keep on pressing. What can you see when you finally remove your elbow?

While doing activity 13.3 you will have noticed that at first you felt pain and discomfort, and you would normally remove your elbow and stop the pain. In order to feel pain, you need nerves to take the *pain message* to the brain and you need to be conscious to receive and interpret the message. Then you need functioning muscles to remove your elbow to prevent any damage to the tissues.

If you had kept on pressing you would have seen the result of direct pressure on the skin where it is covering a bone. When you eventually remove your arm look at the area that was directly under your elbow. At first this area will be paler and feel cool owing to the lack of blood supply, then it will very quickly change colour to look darker and red. Place the back of a bent finger over the area and you should feel heat. This is the effect of the body acknowledging the fact that the specific area has been starved of blood and that it needs oxygen to feed the tissues – hence the increased blood supply. This is called a hyperaemic reaction and is a normal response.

Do not rub the area, as this will only interrupt what nature if trying to do to overcome the effect of prolonged pressure. It has been shown that rubbing an area can actually cause damage to the small blood vessels (capillaries) in the skin. This is also a predisposing factor in the development of a pressure ulcer.

Look again in about 15 minutes to see if the redness and heat have disappeared. The length of time the redness stays is dictated by the length of time the pressure was applied. Should a hyperaemic reaction last longer than an hour then there is a possibility of tissue damage.

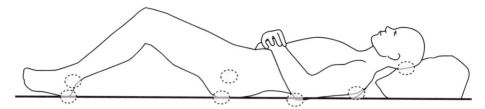

Fig. 13.1   Areas prone to pressure.

When helping a person with their hygiene needs or changing position look at the pressure areas (Fig. 13.1) for any signs of redness and heat. If such signs are present, report them to the registered practitioner, as it could be an indication that the person needs their position changed more frequently.

Activity 13.4

We presume you will have been sitting in more or less the same position for the past half an hour or so while you have been reading. Can you list the parts of you that feel discomfort?

These areas could include:

• Buttocks (sacral area)
• Back of your legs especially if the chair is the wrong size for you

Now lie down on a hard floor on your back without a pillow, if you can bear it. Try to stay there for about five minutes. Consider which parts of your body are now feeling uncomfortable. Your list could include:

• Buttocks (sacral area)
• Shoulder blades (scapulae)
• Head (occipital)
• Heels
• Spine (vertebrae)

Now turn over and lie on your side. What parts of the body feel uncomfortable now? You may include:

• Hip (ischial tuberosity, pelvis)
• Ankle
• Side of your knees
• Shoulder, upper arm
• Ear

Comparing the three lists, you will see that the sacral area (buttocks) is mentioned twice; this is in fact the most common place for a pressure ulcer to develop.

Measures to prevent pressure ulcers

'Prevention is better than cure'. Should a pressure ulcer occur, it can take weeks, even months, to heal, resulting in extreme discomfort and pain to the person. Much has been written on the causes and prevention of pressure ulcers and in this chapter we can only explain the principles. (See Further reading for relevant sources of information.)

If a person has been identified as being at risk of developing a pressure ulcer (usually using a risk assessment tool) due to any number of the factors listed above, a plan of care will be devised and will indicate the actions to be taken to prevent its development. These may include:

- Regular changing of the person's position, at least every two hours. In some people it may need to be more often. It may be advantageous to use a 'turning chart' to record and plan whether the person is on the right or left side, sitting up or lying down etc. The plan can be co-ordinated so that the person is in a suitable position at mealtimes, e.g. sitting up to facilitate eating.
- Using available manual handling equipment to prevent unnecessary friction or shear when moving the person.
- Keeping the skin clean and dry, especially if the person is incontinent, has a high temperature (pyrexia) or is sweating excessively. If the skin is very dry or very moist, special creams may be useful (emollients in bath or cream for dry skin or a barrier cream for moist skin). Do not rub the affected areas as the practice is not recommended[5].
- Bedclothes must be loosely fitted to allow free movement and sheets must not have any creases.
- When attending to personal hygiene needs, the carer must always observe the skin for early signs of the effects of pressure and immediately report any signs of redness or skin abrasion.
- Using special mattresses, pillows and seating cushions that relieve pressure in vulnerable areas.
- Application of special dressings in areas where the skin is sore and liable to breakdown (usually the sacrum and the hip).

In addition to the above it is important that carers pay special attention to the nutritional needs of those in their care, giving assistance with eating and drinking where necessary. Food and fluid intake should be recorded where it is considered necessary and any loss of appetite or lack of motivation to eat or drink should be reported.

Positioning the person

If you are in an uncomfortable position then, as we have already discussed, you will wriggle around to get comfortable. There are times when we as carers will have to position a person when they are unable to do this for themselves.

Relieving pressure is the principal care strategy used in the prevention of pressure ulcers. This is achieved mainly by regular re-positioning and use of appropriate pressure-relieving equipment when necessary.

However, when positioning the person the carer must do so correctly in order to prevent further complications of immobility. By referring to the plan of care we can position the person using soft pillows and any appropriate aids.

When the nervous system is damaged following a stroke or spinal injury or in people who are unconscious or frail and weak, the joints should be positioned within a slightly flexed position to prevent the development of joint contractures. Joint contractures occur when people who are unable to undertake the normal everyday movements develop stiffness in their joints particularly the hip, knee and elbow. As a result they are unable to straighten them. Usually, the person ends up in the foetal position (curled up with their knees bent towards their chest).

Care must be taken to ensure no excess pressure is exerted on the shoulder when the person is on their side in bed. The lower arm and shoulder should be gently eased into position after the person has been turned on their side.

Feet and wrists need to be well supported and bedclothes should be loose to prevent foot and wrist drop. These occur when the limb is positioned incorrectly and the person is unable to adjust their position.

Excess pressure on the calf muscles must be avoided to prevent the development of deep vein thrombosis (DVT). A thrombosis is a clot usually arising in the calf muscles. In people with unaffected mobility, the constant movement of the ankles and feet usually help to pump the blood back to the heart. In a person with impaired mobility this is not always possible and the blood stagnates. In some instances the clot may move up from the leg and lodge in a blood vessel in the lungs. This is known as a pulmonary embolus and is potentially fatal.

Exercise

An important aspect of caring for a person with reduced mobility is exercise. Passive exercises are those that are performed by the carer on behalf of the person. Naturally active exercise, that is, exercise undertaken independently by the person is preferable but in some instances this may not be possible. Passive and active exercise help to prevent some of the possible complications mentioned in the previous section. The physiotherapist plays a major role in this aspect of care and will often advise on the best strategy for each person.

Activity 13.5

While sitting in a chair, raise your left leg and, placing your right hand under your calf, rotate your foot and move it up and down. Can you feel the muscles contracting?

This movement helps to return the blood to the heart and normally occurs when we walk. Immobile persons should therefore undertake some form of foot or ankle exercise at regular intervals.

Further complications of immobility

The immobile client may have many more complications. Some examples are:

- Constipation – due to the lack of exercise and stimulus and/or a change in diet.
- Anorexia – or a general lack of interest in eating and drinking (see Chapter 12 for more detailed coverage of nutrition).
- Calcium movement from the bone – this can occur on long-term bed rest and can lead to kidney stones (renal calculi). It may occur in the client with a spinal injury. The removal of calcium from the bones to the bloodstream will have a weakening effect on the bone (osteoporosis). This could result in bone fracture – usually the neck of femur – and can occur when the client gets out of bed for the first time after a long period of inactivity.
- Depression and frustration – may affect the person because of the change in dependency and lifestyle, resulting in various mood changes. Plans of care should include ways to maintain the person's interest in the family, friends and hobbies. In some care settings, there are 'activities' organisers who help to create a stimulating and pleasant environment.

Activity 13.6

Consider how you can maintain interests, family and friend contacts with your clients.

Your list may include:

- Free access for family and friends
- Daily newspaper available
- Portable telephone with money or card available
- Facilities to read out and reply to letters
- Mobile library visiting the client
- Radio and television at the client's request
- Jigsaws, cards and games
- Knitting and marquetry

This section only covers this vast topic briefly and you should ask around in your own organisation to find out what is available for clients.

Bed making

A comfortable bed is extremely important for the client. Client and individual needs in terms of number of pillows and blankets or duvets must be considered.

Health and safety

See also Chapter 8 on mobility and safe handling of a client.

- Always remember that if a bed has brakes, they must be on.
- If the bed can be raised, bring it up to a safe working height. If the person is in their own home it may be necessary to kneel down to keep your back straight.
- If fire blankets are in use, check these are correctly positioned and attached.

Cross-infection

- Hands must be washed between client/client and plastic aprons should be worn by the carer (see Chapter 9 concerning the control of infection).
- Assess what clean linen is required and only take what is necessary to prevent contamination of clean linen. A linen skip should be close at hand and any linen contaminated with body fluids must be put into the correctly coloured bag (as dictated by local policy).
- Bedclothes should be removed with care to prevent air currents and micro-organisms travelling from one person to another. The bedclothes should be folded neatly onto two chairs or the rack/shelf on the bed, taking care to keep them off the floor.
- Any equipment such as pillows or bed cradles must be placed on a chair near to the client – never on the floor or on someone else's bed.

Principles of bed making

- Careful explanation should be given to the person and their co-operation sought if possible.
- Where possible two people should always make a bed. When making a bed with the person in it their safety and comfort must be maintained at all times.
- Ensure a smooth bottom sheet with no wrinkles or crumbs.
- Bedclothes should be loose enough to allow movement, that is, sheets and blankets should have a tuck put into them to prevent pressure on the toes, heels or ankles (duvets are lighter and allow more movement).
- Pillows should be positioned to give support to the back if the person is sitting up.
- If the person is lying on a special mattress that is connected electrically care must be taken not to interfere with the functioning of the mattress.

Sleep

People spend one third of their lives asleep and this section will discuss why sleep is important for us. It will give an explanation of our normal sleep cycle and how we can assist a client to sleep and rest.

Circadian rhythm

Our daily lives are influenced by our circadian rhythm, which is a daily cycle and our biological clock. A number of factors influence this clock, such as light and dark, and various social cues such as increased traffic noise first thing in the morning. These act as reminders as to the time of the day. They affect our breathing, heart rate, blood pressure and bowel activity.

During the *day* we are actively moving about, eating and using energy. Our body prepares for this by producing hormones (adrenaline and steroids) that help to keep us awake and alert; this is very much influenced by light. Our blood pressure and pulse rise during the day, reaching their maximum between 12.00 and 18.00 hours, while our temperature is at its maximum between 18.00 and 24.00 hours.

During the *evening* our adrenaline levels fall and we begin to find it more difficult to concentrate as our body is preparing for sleep both mentally and physically.

During the *night* the body and mind rest and sleep, with the blood pressure, pulse and temperature being lowest between 02.00 and 06.00 hours. It is during this time of inactivity that growth and repair of tissues such as skin, bone and bone marrow are thought to take place.

Early morning, from about 04.00 hours, the body prepares for activity and adrenaline is produced.

Should our normal routine and sleep patterns change, this will have an effect on us. Being a client in hospital causes disruption to circadian rhythms due to changes in light and dark cues, imposed meal and sleep times and changes in rituals. Similarly, nurses' working shifts can be disrupted and can take seven days to re-adjust. The effects are similar to jet lag. People complain of fatigue, sleep problems, headaches, indigestion, reduced appetite and bowel problems[6].

Importance of sleep

Sleep is something we all need and there are many theories about why we need it, although much about it is not fully understood. Sleep is affected by thoughts, emotions and the amount of stimulation as well as chemicals and hormones (serotonin). Growth hormone is released as we sleep. There is also a link between sleep and the immune system (sleep deprivation will reduce our resistance to disease).

Activity 13.7

Make a list of the reasons why you feel sleep is important.

Your list may include:

- The brain needs time for a rest in order to sweep away unnecessary memories and consolidate learning.
- The body needs time to rest, and sleep has a restorative function.
- Sleep aids the process of healing wounds and tissue repair.
- Sleep and rest make us feel better.

You may find it easier to identify what happens to us if we do not get enough sleep (i.e. sleep deprivation).

Activity 13.8

Make a list of the effects of sleep deprivation.

Your list may include:

- Difficult to co-ordinate and focus your eyes
- Not being able to concentrate
- Being lethargic
- Being anti-social
- Feeling tired, which could lead to chronic fatigue
- Feeling cold
- Pain feels worse
- Being irritable and restless
- Increase in stress levels
- Becoming depressed
- Feeling slightly confused
- Having micro-sleeps

You have probably have felt these effects yourself and you will certainly have seen them in others.

Time spent in sleep

We spend up to a third of our lives asleep and the length of our sleep periods changes throughout our lives (Fig. 13.2). This is of course individual and can depend on culture and habits. Many prime ministers in the past have managed on very little sleep, less than four hours a night, while others had a longer sleep plus a nap in the afternoon.

Baby
16 out of 24 hours

Teenager
10–11 hours a night

Adult
7 hours a night

Older people
5–7 hours a night plus naps during the day

Fig. 13.2 Time spent in sleep.

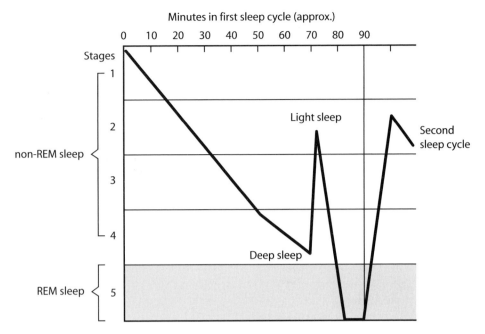

Fig. 13.3   The sleep cycle. REM, rapid eye movement (used with permission from Roper *et al.*)[13].

The sleep cycle

There are two types of sleep: non-REM (no rapid eye movement) and REM (rapid eye movement). Non-REM sleep has four different stages in cycles, going from light to deep sleep and then the sequence reverses, going from deep to light sleep. REM sleep comes at the end of each sleep cycle and is a much lighter sleep, during which the eyes move rapidly from side to side below the closed eyelids (Fig. 13.3). It is during this stage that dreams occur. The person moves about and changes position and any snoring may cease.

A complete sleep cycle lasts about 90 minutes and is repeated about four or five times during an average eight-hour night's sleep. Therefore, a full cycle could be stages 1 to 4, then 4 to 1 with REM sleep between each cycle (see Fig. 13.3). As you fall asleep the brain becomes less responsive to outside stimuli and the body relaxes.

Non-REM sleep

Stage 1

This is when you fall asleep. The body begins to relax and all the vital signs (temperature, pulse, respiration and blood pressure) are normal. The person can be easily awoken at this time. This stage lasts about 20 minutes. If it lasts more than 40 minutes then the individual is thought to be suffering from insomnia. If awakened, people feel as though they have been daydreaming.

Stage 2

This is a period of light sleep, when brain activity begins to slow down. The person can be easily aroused.

Stage 3

The muscles become relaxed and the vital signs become depressed as sleep becomes heavier. The sleeping person is difficult to arouse and rarely moves.

Stage 4

During this stage of deep sleep, arousal is difficult; the vital signs are at their lowest. However, the digestive tract is very active during this stage. Sleepwalking may occur. This stage of deep sleep is reduced in older people. It is believed to be responsible for restoring and resting the body.

REM sleep

This is a much lighter sleep and can last from five to 15 minutes. It occurs at the end of each cycle, i.e. after the final stage 1 sleep of one cycle and before the initial stage 1 sleep of the next cycle. The blood flow to the brain increases and the person dreams and moves about more. This stage is thought to be necessary to restore us mentally and emotionally. Although we do not always remember our dreams, we all do dream and you may well be aware of them should you wake up during this stage. We tend to consolidate our learning during this stage.[7] Children's growth is at its maximum when they are asleep at night. Growth hormone is released at this time and can act because adrenaline and steroid levels are low. Sleep during the day does not have the same effect. Similarly, wounds/injuries in adults heal best when asleep at night.

Factors that influence sleep

Activity 13.9

List some activities that could induce sleep.

Your list could include:

- Having a hot milky drink or snack
- Reading
- Having a warm bath to relax
- Keeping to a certain routine
- Listening to music
- Praying or meditating

- Dimming the lights
- Sexual activity

Admission to hospital and changes to lifestyle may alter sleep patterns.

Change in routine

Routines change when people enter some sort of communal life and it can be difficult to meet everyone's individual needs. During our life we become conditioned in our preparation to go to sleep, our brain learns this from an early age. For instance, keeping to the same routine for a child is important to induce sleep and if the normal bedtime story is missed, the child may find it difficult to go to sleep. Keeping to a routine of specific behaviour informs the brain that we are getting ready for bed and these messages are relayed to other parts of the brain and body, inducing sleep.

It is important to find out how long a client normally sleeps, what time they go to bed and what routine they follow before going to sleep. Adapting their care to comply with their normal routine as much as possible will not only make the client feel more secure in the environment, but will help them go to sleep. This will help overcome initial insomnia, which occurs at sleep onset; racing mind phenomena or anxiety will make this type of insomnia worse.

A substance called tryptophan, which is found in milk, beef and beans, is thought to promote sleep onset, while 500mg caffeine, equivalent to three cups of coffee drunk over 24 hours, can disrupt sleep. Nicotine, soda water, alcohol and some medications can also disrupt sleep patterns.

Sleep can be reduced by 20–25% when a client goes into hospital, yet the need for sleep increases with illness and stress. I am sure that you have experienced a client complaining of lack of sleep while in hospital, and looking forward to going home for a good night's sleep!

Activity 13.10

List anything that could prevent someone sleeping in hospital.

Your list could include:

- Noise from people talking, telephones, televisions
- Noise outside the ward area
- People moving about with noisy shoes
- Squeaky equipment and machines
- Pain and discomfort
- Anxiety
- Bladder distension
- Difficulty in breathing
- Change in surroundings

- Unfamiliar noises and lights, and the close proximity of other people
- Strange bed and bedding
- Room too hot and stuffy or too cold
- Being either linked to monitoring equipment or in close proximity to someone else
- Confused and ill clients nearby requiring care
- Settling the ward late and waking people early

How can we help promote sleep?

Reduce pain and promote comfort

This topic is considered in more depth in the next section concerning pain. The main principles we should consider are listed here:

- Sometimes by changing position and using a supportive mattress and pillows, a client can be made more comfortable.
- Massage can relax a client and, used in conjunction with aromatherapy, can reduce anxiety and induce sleep.
- Analgesics should be administered to control pain, and maintenance doses should be given before the client complains of severe pain. It is important to monitor and evaluate the level of pain and the effect of analgesics.
- A full bladder or fear of being incontinent will prevent restful sleep. Always ensure a client has had the opportunity to pass urine before settling down to sleep and be prepared for the client waking in the night to pass urine. It is essential for a client to have a means of attracting a carer's attention during the night. For the ambulant client, positioning of the bed near to a toilet or a commode will reduce the incidence of falls.

Reduce anxiety and stress

Anyone in a new environment will be anxious owing to concern over their illness or to separation from their family, friends or a pet. This anxiety stimulates the body and prevents sleep. We all need information and fear of the unknown is an obvious cause of stress. The following may help reduce anxiety and stress:

- Spending time listening to and talking with a client is very supportive and can help someone to settle down to sleep. Clients with sleeping problems need to be shown both empathy and understanding.
- Relaxation by listening to music or reading may help to induce sleep; however, for some clients these may act as stimuli and raise the arousal level and inhibit the onset of sleep.
- Allowing visitors to stay with a client as they settle down to sleep may be beneficial. Providing a client with access to a telephone so they can chat to their family is also very helpful.

Aid breathing and help to prevent gastro-oesophageal reflux (indigestion)

If a client is helped into a more upright position this may facilitate breathing and help control reflux (when the contents of the stomach pass up the oesophagus).

Activity 13.11

Consider how you would know if a client had slept well.

You could ask the client about the following:

- How long did it take them to fall asleep?
- How many times do they remember waking up?
- What sort of things woke them up?
- How long did it take them to get back to sleep?
- What time did they awake and not return to sleep?
- How long did they sleep in total?
- It is a very personal judgement and not related to how much sleep they appear to have had.

Reduce noise level

We are not always aware of the level of noise around a client. As we grow older we become more sensitive to noise. Consider how a young baby, once they are off to sleep, can sleep through door bells ringing, radio and television; an older person, however, quickly wakes up if they hear an unfamiliar sound. We need to consider this fact when caring for older people and ensure the care environment is quiet and conducive to sleep. Fox found that noise was the main reason for clients taking sleeping tablets while in hospital[8].

Some of these causes may be out of our control, but if we prepare the client by explaining the cause of the noise, it may help them to accept it and so cope better. We should be aware that although we need stimuli to keep us awake and alert during the night, the client does not, so we must make an effort to reduce the noise level in the care area[9].

Light

Light is a stimulant and it acts on our brain and tells us that we should be awake and alert. It also makes the body produce hormones that enable us to be active (think of the sun waking you up in the morning).

It may be beneficial for a client to have some sort of night light on, or a light switch nearby, as it enables them to orientate themselves to a new environment or ensures that they can find their way around a familiar one and avoid falls.

Temperature of the environment

The temperature needs to be warm but not stuffy; an ideal temperature is about 20 °C. There also needs to be an adequate amount of fresh air to promote sleep. As we grow older our temperature control mechanism tends to diminish. As our body temperature drops during sleep it is important to maintain a constant ambient temperature of 21 °C for older people and ensure they have light but warm nightclothes and bedclothes.

Nursing interventions

The more critically ill or dependent a client is, the more they are disturbed during the night and are unable to complete a normal sleep cycle. This can lead to sleep deprivation, resulting in possible confusion and, in the case of a surgical client, a delay in wound healing. Care needs to be planned with as little disturbance as possible. This can be achieved by only giving essential care to a client during the night or clustering activities together so they may complete a full 90-minute sleep cycle. Nurses should also seek out clients who are not sleeping and find out what their individual problem is[10].

Clients in hospital are very dependent on the nurse controlling the environment and considering their comfort needs. Without this their recovery may be delayed.

Pain

Caring for clients in pain can be challenging, especially emotionally. Pain is an individual, unique experience and we can never make assumptions about the pain a client is experiencing. Although two clients may have the same operation, this does not mean they will experience the same amount of pain. It is often easy to say: 'Mr Smith is up and around now but Mr Bloggs is not so he must be making a fuss.'

McCaffery[11] states: 'Pain is whatever the experiencing person says it is, and exists whenever he says it does.' This definition is useful for two reasons as it highlights the importance of asking the client about their pain and the importance of believing what they say. If the client does not feel believed, this will affect their relationship with their carers. Good communication and trust are essential for successful pain management.

What is pain?

> **Activity 13.12**
>
> What is pain? This may seem like a simple question. Spend some time writing down your thoughts.

You may have noted some of the body's way of telling you that something is wrong:

- Warning sign, e.g. pain or swelling
- Sign to show things are getting worse

- Response to injury – inflammation – pain, heat, swelling, loss of function
- Unpleasant feeling/experience
- Sign that shows you are healing – pain, swelling, heat resolve and function returns
- Sensation to prevent movement and stop you doing further harm (See Chapter 9, Fig. 9.4)

You may have had more, all of which may be correct, because pain means different things to different people. Another useful definition of pain is 'an unpleasant sensory and emotional experience in association with actual or potential tissue damage, or described in terms of such damage'[12].

Sometimes people experience pain and there is no obvious physical cause; this does not mean the pain is not real. Likewise, there are people who have walked miles from an accident on a broken leg to get help, yet felt no pain at the time!

The pain message

Activity 13.13

When you last stubbed your toe or trapped your finger what did you do?

In your answer, you may have included:

- Rubbed it
- Screamed
- Swore
- Jumped up and down
- Shouted

On the other hand, perhaps you did nothing until a time that was more convenient!

So how does the pain message reach the brain? We have nerve fibres all over the body which, when injury occurs start to send a message. This message travels along the nerve and we often refer to this as a pathway. This message continues along the pathway to the spinal cord then up to the brain. At the point where the message enters the spinal cord is an area we call the 'gate'. If the gate is closed this stops the pain message travelling up the spinal cord, and hence the brain does not receive the message of pain. When the gate is open, this allows the pain message to travel along the spinal cord, thus reaching the brain. The brain then tells us we are in pain and we react or behave in a way that may be the same as other people or individual to us (Fig. 13.4).

Other messages like touch also travel along the same pathway that the pain message uses. If these two messages try to use the pathway at the same time i.e. pain and touch, only so much of either can get through. This explains why rubbing an area lessens the pain temporarily.

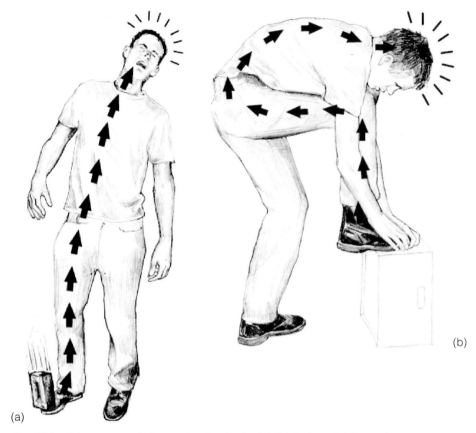

Fig. 13.4   Pain message being sent to the brain. (a) Brick drop. (b) Foot rub.

There is one further important fact to consider. Our brain interprets the pain message, and it is also capable of stopping the pain message. We do this in two ways. We may ignore the message, which allows us to act normally, for example walking on a broken leg to get help. Alternatively, we may send a second message from the brain down the spinal cord that blocks our original pain message. Hypnosis and relaxation probably work in this way. This also demonstrates the importance of our state of mind in controlling and tolerating pain. However, this is only a part of the picture and it is not just a case of 'mind over matter'.

How do we know a client is in pain?

The best way of finding out if a client is in pain is to ask them. Asking the client is the first step in understanding what the client's pain is like and beginning to help relieve it. Of course, some clients may not be able to tell you that they are in pain.

Activity 13.14

How might you know a client was in pain if they were unable to tell you?

You may have come up with the following suggestions:

- Facial expression
- Hunched up
- Rubbing
- Crying
- Moaning
- Sweating
- Clammy
- Pale
- Reduced appetite
- Being sick
- Being quiet
- Raised pulse

It is important to remember that if the pain has continued for a long time many of the above signs may not be present. Clients who have had long-term pain may appear on the surface to be pain free. Do not assume this is the case.

We tend to assume that clients will tell us if they have pain and need a painkiller. However, clients may expect us to know when they are in pain without their having to tell us.

Factors that affect the way individuals respond to pain

Family influence

The way an adult responds to pain may relate to their childhood experiences. For example if a hurt child cries he or she may be cuddled or alternatively may be ignored and praised when they stop crying.

Social influence

The response of others to our complaints of pain may affect the way we behave.

Cultural influence

There has been much research into the influences of culture on a person's responses to pain. It appears people from some cultures may prefer to be alone when in pain and others prefer company. Perhaps more importantly, some cultures do not express their pain through words (stiff upper lip) while others are used to expressing their pain more loudly.

It is important to remember that none of the examples above means an individual is making a fuss or has no pain.

Language

A language barrier can prevent clients from telling you they have pain. Being unable to express pain may result in fear and uncertainty. It is particularly important to ask a client about pain, either through the family or through an interpreter.

Part of the body

A client may find it hard to talk about some areas of their body.

Acute and chronic pain

Now we have thought about how we experience pain, we can look at two broad categories of pain: acute and chronic.

Acute pain

Several features define pain as acute:

- It usually persists for a short length of time.
- It is often associated with healing, for example following surgery or injury.
- It is expected to go when healing is complete.

Chronic pain

Chronic pain is associated with different features:

- It is usually prolonged (more than three months).
- It often gets worse.
- It is often associated with deteriorating problem(s).
- It is associated with changes in lifestyle, personality and a reduced ability to carry out day-to-day activities.

Activity 13.15

Write two headings, one called acute pain and one called chronic pain. Under each heading, give examples of the causes of each type of pain.

Here are some examples:

Acute pain

- Sudden injury
- Appendicitis
- Headache
- Toothache

Chronic pain

- Backache
- Arthritis
- Cancer pain

Sometimes an acute pain can become chronic if it persists and the underlying cause is not treated. Occasionally with chronic pain, there is no obvious physical cause but this does not mean the pain is any less real.

Pain-killing drugs (analgesics)

The reason for giving pain-killing drugs is different for the two categories of pain. For acute pain, the aim is to give pain-killing drugs for a short time and then to reduce and stop them quickly as the pain improves. For chronic pain, we often have to give strong analgesics such as morphine. Often the dose is increased regularly. We also give these analgesics to keep the pain away and the client pain-free.

There are many different analgesics and for clients in pain we usually follow the guidelines shown in Fig. 13.5 and move up the analgesic ladder until we reach a drug that works.

Routes of administration

There are several different ways of giving analgesic drugs:

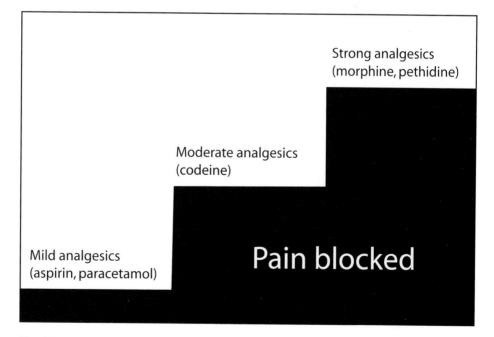

Fig. 13.5 Analgesics work by blocking the pain message.

- In tablet form (orally), depending on the drug
- By injection (subcutaneously, intramuscularly, intravenously) administered either in single dose, a does at regular intervals or by a pump which gives a continuous dose or is controlled by the client
- By a gas, commonly used at the scene of accidents and during childbirth
- By suppository

Activity 13.16

What alternative methods might we use to control pain other than medicines?

You may have thought of the following:

- Gentle rubbing or massage (not bony areas or pressure areas, check with the person in charge first): touch
- Changing position: physical comfort
- Making client comfortable: physical comfort
- Talking to them: mental comfort
- Relaxation: mental comfort
- Diversion, e.g. music, art: mental comfort
- Just being with them: mental comfort

There are some other methods, which come under the heading of complementary therapies, such as aromatherapy, hypnosis, reflexology and acupuncture. The use of complementary therapies to help relieve pain is increasing.

Pain threshold

The pain threshold is the limit to which the individual can tolerate pain before it becomes unacceptable. The pain threshold is unique to the individual and the individual's state of mind can alter the pain threshold. It is therefore something we can help to increase and hence ease distress. A high pain threshold is not a virtue and nor is high pain tolerance; they are individual responses that may charge according to the circumstance.

Activity 13.17

What factors do you think would lower or raise the pain threshold?

Under lowering the pain threshold (lower tolerance of pain) you may have included:

- Fear
- Stress

- Uncertainty
- Discomfort
- Anger
- Sadness
- Anxiety
- Lack of sleep
- Being isolated
- Lack of support

Under raising the pain threshold (higher tolerance to pain) you may have included:

- Sleep
- Low stress
- Being kept informed
- Creative activity
- Companionship
- Being happy
- Low anxiety
- Relief of other symptoms
- Comfortable
- Support

The role of the carer in pain control

We have covered a great deal of ground on the topic of pain. It is now time to consider the carer's role in the management of pain.

Clients may experience acute or chronic pain. In both cases, the client can expect to become pain-free. It may sometimes take a short time to find the appropriate analgesic and dose.

It is important to check whether a particular drug is not working. Most drugs will take effect within half an hour of their administration. Speedy reporting allows the client to become pain-free more quickly and alerts staff to the fact that a drug is not working. We also discussed how we might know if a client was in pain but cannot tell us and again this needs observing and reporting.

As carers, we may offer many of the comforting actions discussed under the section on alternative methods of pain control, such as relaxation, distraction and change of position.

In the section on the pain threshold, we discussed how we might raise clients' tolerance to pain and ease their distress. Again, the carer can perform many of these actions for example reassurance, company if required and support. If necessary find someone who can give the client the information they need.

Finally, it is most important never to judge the client but to continue with an individual approach to care. The client knows their own pain best but we can help support them. To manage pain well the carer requires good communication skills and to try to understand the client's pain from their point of view.

Summary

In this chapter we have considered rest, comfort and pain control for the client. The causes and prevention of pressure ulcers were explained and advice given on how to maintain the comfort of a client confined to bed or with limited mobility. We hope it has given you an insight into the importance of maintaining movement and the prevention of pressure ulcers, considering not only the physical aspects of care but also the psychological.

The final section considered the pain pathway and the other messages that use the same pathway, such as touch. Finally, we considered the state of mind of the client and the role of the carer.

References

1. Dealey, C. (1999) *The Care of Wounds*, 2nd edition. Blackwell, London.
2. Collins, F. (2001) Repositioning to prevent pressure sores – what is the evidence? *Nursing Standard* **15** (22), 54–56.
3. Casey, G. (1998) The importance of nutrition in wound healing. *Nursing Standard* **13** (3), 51–56.
4. Clay, M. (2000) Pressure sore prevention in nursing homes. *Nursing Standard* **14** (44), 45–50.
5. European Pressure Ulcer Advisory Panel Guidelines (1998) A policy statement on the prevention of pressure ulcers from the European Pressure Ulcer Advisory Panel. *British Journal of Nursing* **7** (15), 888, 890.
6. Humm, C. (2000) A hard day's night. *Nursing Times* **96** (20), 28–31.
7. Howcroft, D. and Jones, R. (1999) Sleep, older people and dementia. *Nursing Times* **95** (33), 54–56.
8. Fox, M.R. (1999) The importance of sleep. *Nursing Standard* **13** (24), 44–47.
9. Meredith, R.E. (2000) Improving the quality of care provided at night. *Professional Nurse* **15** (8), 502–505.
10. Wilkinson, J. (2000) All for a quiet night. *Nursing Standard* **14** (33), 25.
11. McCaffery, M. (1968) *Nursing Practice Theories Relating to Cognition, Bodily Pain, and Man – Environment Interactions*. University of California, Los Angeles, USA.
12. Twycross, R. and Wilcox, A. (2001) *Symptom Control in Advanced Cancer*, 3rd edition. Radcliffe Medical Press, Oxford.
13. Roper, N., Logan, W., Tierney, A.J. and Holland, K. (1996) *The Elements of Nursing a Model Based on a Model of Living*, 4th edition. Churchill Livingstone, Edinburgh.

Further reading

Davis, B. (1999) *Caring for People in Pain*. Routledge, London.
Hogg, G. (1998) Sleep deprivation in a high dependency unit. *Professional Nurse* **13** (10), 693–696.
National Institute for Clinical Excellence (2001) *Pressure Ulcer Risk Assessment and Prevention Clinical Guideline*. National Institute for Clinical Excellence, London.
Royal College of Nursing (2000) *Pressure Ulcer Risk Assessment and Prevention – Clinical Practice Guidelines*. Royal College of Nursing, London.

Chapter 14

Postnatal care

Rebecca Sutton and Dorothy Stables*

Overview

This chapter will help you to understand the postnatal period, the way you can contribute to the care of mothers and babies in the days after childbirth, and how to help the new mother to develop her parenting skills.

Key words: Puerperium; postnatal period; postnatal care of mothers; of babies; physical care; emotional care; infant feeding; artificial feeding; breast-feeding; midwife's role; parenting

---

Activity 14.1

Before reading this chapter consider:

- if you have children – how it was shortly after they were born? From what help or advice did you benefit in the early days?

Or

- if you do not have children – ask friends and family what help or advice was, or would have been, useful to them.

There are no exact answers, but spending a little time thinking of these issues will help you with the subject.

Puerperium

The puerperium, also called the postnatal period, is the time that begins immediately after the birth of the baby and placenta (afterbirth) and lasts for six weeks after delivery. The placenta is attached to the uterine wall and to the fetus by the umbilical cord. It is the means by which oxygen and nourishment pass from the mother to the fetus. Impediments to the vital supplies can harm the unborn baby. The peuperium is the period when great physical and psychological changes

---

*Contributor to the original version of this chapter in the first edition.

occur within the woman's body as it returns to normal. During this time the woman may have to adjust to her new role as a mother and learn how to care for herself and her new baby. Several health professionals are responsible for the care provided to women during this important period of time. As well as your-self, other professionals involved include the midwife, the health visitor and the general practitioner (GP).

Role of the midwife

The midwife is responsible for the care of the woman and baby in the postnatal period in both hospital and community settings, having also provided care for her during the antenatal period and childbirth. Since April 2002, the Nursing and Midwifery Council (NMC) has been overseeing midwifery practice. Up until then, it had been the United Kingdom Central Council for Nursing, Midwifery and Health Visiting (UKCC) which had been responsible for this duty. The UKCC published *The Midwives' Rules and Code of Professional Conduct* in 1998[1]; at the time of writing this still serves as the guidelines for midwifery practice. One such guideline within *The Midwives' Rules* has defined the time period for a midwife to provide postnatal care to a woman and baby as: 'A period of not less than 10 days and not more than 28 days after the end of labour during which the con-tinued attendance of a midwife on the mother and baby is requisite.' Thus the midwife must provide at least 10 days of care of mothers and babies. If there have been complications, for example illness of either mother or baby, then mid-wifery care should continue for up to 28 days.

Role of the health care assistant

A health care assistant (HCA) provides support to both women and midwives and should support the advice given to the woman by her midwife. An HCA helps the woman with day-to-day care, and she may be the first person to pick up any problems with either the mother or the baby.

Role of the health visitor

Health visitors start visiting new mothers and their babies from 11 days after the delivery, to check on how the baby is developing and growing. They also see how the mother is adapting at home with her new baby. Health visitors offer advice on matters relating to maternal health, nutrition for a growing baby – for example, weaning from milk to solids at an appropriate age, vaccinations and issues which may arise over the following months and years. They will check regularly on both mother and baby until the child is 5 years old, either in a specific clinic at a GP's surgery or in the family home.

Role of the GP

The GP provides a six-week check for both mother and baby. This is to ensure that the mother's body has returned to normal after delivery, to provide contraceptive advice, to check the baby regarding his or her growth and development and to advise on initial vaccinations. If any complications arise, usually medical complications, with the mother during the antenatal, labour or postnatal periods, she may be referred to a consultant obstetrician for her postnatal check, to determine whether her health is improving and perhaps provide a plan of care for her next delivery.

Understanding the changes

You need to be aware of what is normal in both the newly delivered mother and baby. Both of their bodies are undergoing changes and you should be able to recognise what is or is not usual so that you can alert the responsible professional, normally the midwife, to any potential problem.

Changes in the mother's body following birth

During pregnancy, a mother's body changes considerably as it adapts to help the baby grow and develop safely. Once the baby has been born further changes occur in several of the organs of the mother's body. These changes enable the body to return to normal and in the case of the breasts to provide food for the baby, the most dramatic changes happening within the first ten days after delivery. The organs experiencing the most changes are the breasts, the uterus, kidneys and legs.

Breasts

Breasts are the mammary glands, normally two in number, which are situated on the front of the chest wall and are separated from the chest wall by a layer of loose connective tissue. Following delivery, you may notice significant changes in the breasts. Immediately after birth they will start producing colostrum, which will be followed a few days later by engorged (full and heavy) breasts as milk is produced. This will be discussed in more detail below.

Uterus

The uterus, also called the womb, is a pear-shaped, hollow, muscular organ situated in the pelvis between the bladder and the rectum. In the puerperium, the uterus slowly returns to the near-normal pre-pregnancy size, achieved by a process called involution. Most involution occurs during the first ten days after delivery, followed by a gradual return to normal over the next six weeks. Within these first few days, with the uterus beginning to return to normal, some mothers experience period-like pains, which are called 'after-pains'. These pains can also occur during breast-feeding because a hormone released to help expel the milk during feeding also helps cause the uterus to contract. Such after-pains are usually felt more by women who have had more than one baby.

Lochia

Lochia is the normal vaginal loss that women experience after delivery. In the first few days this is like a heavy period, gradually decreasing over the following days. The lochia pass through three stages within the first 10–14 days after delivery. These stages are called rubra, serosa and alba. Rubra is similar to a heavy period and occurs from after delivery of the placenta to day three. This then changes to serosa at about day four until around day seven. It is brownish in colour. Finally, alba, which is pinkish in colour, first occurs between days eight and ten. Mothers may experience vaginal loss for up to six weeks after delivery and should be encouraged to use sanitary towels rather than tampons as the latter may introduce infection or impede healing. The lochia has a distinctive odour but this should not be offensive.

If the lochia is offensive, there may be several causes, for example poor hygiene or infection. If the woman reports that she is passing clots or is bleeding heavily keep any used sanitary towels and any clots that she may have passed. If a clot has been passed, it is important to ascertain the size and to show it to a midwife, particularly if the clot is the size of a 50-pence piece or larger. Women occasionally pass small stringy clots, which may be normal, but still inform a midwife if these occur. There are a number of reasons why a woman may pass a clot: retained products, trauma (for example if the woman has had a tear) or may be due to 'pooling'. Pooling occurs when the mother has been lying down for a period of time and has just got up. It is still important to inform the midwife of any clots passed, if the lochia appears heavy or if you or the mother have any concerns.

Kidneys and bladder

The kidneys are two bean-shaped organs situated in the upper abdomen towards the back. The bladder, the 'reservoir for urine', is situated in the pelvis. It is important to determine the amount of urine passed after delivery, as in the last trimester (the last third) of pregnancy women pass small amounts of urine but frequently. This is because the capacity of the bladder is reduced, there being a heavy uterus on it. Once the baby has been born, the woman will pass a normal amount of urine, usually between 200 ml and 300 ml. Some women may experience pain on micturition (urinating or passing water), which may be due to several factors, including perineal trauma such as a tear or infection. If this occurs advise the woman to increase her fluid intake, particularly water or certain fruit juices, for example cranberry or grapefruit juice. Since urine contains acid the extra fluid helps reduce the acidity of the urine. If the woman does experience pain, inform the midwife. If she has a urinary tract infection it will need to be treated. Also inform the midwife should the woman feel that she is frequently passing small amounts of urine, as this may be another sign of infection. Women occasionally find themselves unable to pass urine, which can be accompanied by lower abdominal pain. If this occurs, inform the midwife immediately as this may require catheterisation.

Legs

The legs may become swollen following delivery and this is normal. Mothers should be reassured of this accordingly and encouraged to mobilise and to perform ankle exercises. The swelling (called oedema) is caused by an increase in fluid within the tissue of the lower limbs. Movement helps the fluid return to the blood supply.

It is important to observe the mother's legs after delivery for any signs of heat, stiffness or even cramp-like pain, as any of these may be a sign of deep vein thrombosis (DVT). If a mother reports any of these signs, report them to a midwife who then may contact a doctor who can initiate treatment. A DVT is a blood clot occurring in veins within the legs. This can be a potentially life-threatening condition as a clot can break off and end up in the lungs. A clot in the lungs, called pulmonary embolism, can block the flow of blood to the heart. Women who are most at risk of DVT may be those women who are least mobile – for example, those who have had a caesarean or an epidural.

Activity 14.2

Make a list of potential signs of problems with the newly delivered mother's health that you should report to the midwife.

Hormones and periods

A woman's next period after childbirth will not occur immediately. The hormones, progesterone and oestrogen, that control the menstrual cycle (how often periods occur) have just started to return to normal. The level of progesterone, which increased during pregnancy, has, now that pregnancy has ended, suddenly dropped and may take a while to return to its pre-pregnancy fluctuating level. However, it is possible for a woman to ovulate within 3 weeks of delivery, so she can become pregnant again very quickly. The midwife will have advised the mother of this.

Changes in the emotional state of new mothers

Once a woman has had a baby, she may initially feel elated when her baby is in her arms. In some cases, however, a woman's emotions may take her on what, for her, feels like a rollercoaster and she may experience a certain amount of anxiety or depression alternating with feelings of elation. A new mother may also feel tired, irritable and unsure of herself. She may have a number of concerns, for example that her baby is not feeding well, particularly if the baby is breast-feeding. She may watch her baby while she or he is sleeping to ensure that her baby is alive and subsequently may not rest properly between feeds. If any of these concerns arise, reassure and support the woman – and her partner, if he is present, as he may have concerns as well – and inform the midwife of any concerns that you or the mother may have.

Between days two and five, a number of mothers can become quite tearful and may cry over what may appear to be the smallest thing. This is called the 'baby blues', with mothers needing support and reassurance that this is perfectly normal. It usually resolves about 24–48 hours later. This condition is thought to be caused by changes in a mother's hormonal levels after delivery. Encourage mothers to rest when they can, as this again helps with healing and, in some cases, with their emotional state.

The blues are different from postnatal depression which may occur from about 14 days postnatally and, also, puerperal psychosis which can occur at any time following delivery. If a woman becomes depressed her expression may appear lifeless and she may appear low emotionally. Puerperal psychosis is a much rarer but different condition with women behaving strangely, having hallucinations or delusions. If you notice that the woman is depressed or behaving strangely, then inform the midwife.

Although you need to be aware of these conditions, they are exceptional: as Niven has noted, the majority of women tend to cope 'remarkably well' because they are 'highly motivated' in caring for a new-born baby.[2]

Postnatal care of the mother

Observations

Observations are an important part of postnatal care, and it will depend on the unit you work in as to whether you perform these. If so, they will be taught in your clinical area and you may learn how to take a woman's pulse, temperature and blood pressure. The normal range of pulse rate is between 60 beats and 80 beats per minute. The normal range of the temperature is between 36.2 °C and 37.2 °C with normal blood pressure being between 90/50 mmHg and 120/80 mmHg.

The pulse and temperature are indicators of whether a mother is developing an infection. Blood pressure may be an indicator of several things – for example, it may be raised if the woman is in pain or is developing a condition called pre-eclampsia or lowered if the woman is losing blood. If you have taken the observations it is important that they are documented accurately and if there any deviations from normal, inform the midwife.

Personal hygiene

Women who have had vaginal deliveries, for example a normal or ventouse delivery, are usually independent in their care, for example in washing, walking around and beginning to look after their babies. In a few cases new mothers may need a little encouragement in general cleanliness for both themselves and their babies. Use care and tact when bringing the subject up and provide support, education and reassurance if required.

After delivery and despite a blood loss, mothers may take a shower or a bath, which should help them to feel refreshed and 'normal'. Depending upon the policy of the unit you work in, women who have had a caesarean section can be offered a bed-bath within the first 24 hours, as within this initial period they are not very mobile. After this, they may be more mobile and can have a shower or bath if they wish, depending upon your unit's policy. Women who have had a vaginal delivery may take a shower or bath sooner if they wish.

If a mother has a wound, from a caesarean section or a tear or episiotomy on her perineum ('down below' – the area between her vagina and anus), advise her to keep the affected area clean and to dry carefully. If the woman does have stitches 'down below', also advise her to change her pads regularly.

Nutritional needs of mothers in the postnatal period

After delivery, all women should eat a well-balanced, healthy diet. The nutritional requirements of women who are breast-feeding increase by approximately 25%. Most hospitals have a menu that varies daily. The menu aims to offer a healthy diet. Bear in mind that some women may have difficulty understanding the menu, so they may need help in filling the menu-request in. Some may have specific dietary needs, either because of a medical condition such as diabetes or because they are vegetarian, so be aware of and sympathetic to a woman's dietary needs. The type of delivery and when a woman delivered may also determine what she can eat and when, for example immediately after a caesarean section. If this is the case, do check with the midwife looking after the woman to see what she can eat.

Activity 14.3

Think about mothers from different cultural backgrounds. Can you think of any other needs such a mother may have and other methods you could utilise to help care for her?

Changes in the baby

Once born, a baby's adaptation to extra-uterine life involves a number of systems including:

- The baby's lungs' having to inflate to enable the baby to start breathing
- Circulatory changes allowing the baby to obtain oxygen from his or her own lungs rather than the placenta
- The baby needing to regulate his or her own body temperature

- The baby's own immune system beginning to help fight infection
- Use of the gastro-intestinal system to ingest food and for its excretion

Recognising the normal appearance and behaviour of the baby

One of the midwives' duties is examination of the new-born shortly after birth to determine whether the baby has any problems and have them treated accordingly. She will perform a top-to-toe examination to ensure that the baby is normal, which includes:

- Birth weight – should be between 2.5 kg and 4.5 kg
- Length – should be approximately 52 cm
- Skin colour – should be healthy and free from yellow, grey or blue
- Abdomen – should be round in shape
- Muscle tone – how the baby moves and holds the position of his or her limbs
- Respiratory rate – should be between 35 and 60 breaths per minute, although this may appear variable with the baby having a strong cry

The midwife will also examine the baby's fontanelle (soft spot on the top of the head), the spine and genitalia to ensure that all is well.

Examining and caring for the baby

If you are caring for the baby, for example if you are either helping the mother with the baby's care or if the mother is temporarily unavailable, you become responsible for him or her. Therefore, if you detect any deviation from normal either in the baby's appearance or behaviour, if you notice any change within the baby's condition, inform the midwife as soon as possible.

When you are caring for a baby observe his or her condition, for example the colour, temperature, breathing rate and behaviour.

If you notice the baby's skin or the whites of the baby's eyes have taken on a yellow hue, inform a midwife as soon as possible. When a baby goes yellow, this is a condition called jaundice and occurs in about 50% of babies over 24 hours of age. When a baby has jaundice it is important that the baby is fed regularly, as this can help treat the jaundice, as can placing the baby next to a non-draughty window.

A safe, warm environment needs to be maintained for baby. Help new mums in achieving this. It can be done by showing how to dress and wrap a baby. This also occurs when you bathe a baby, as a baby needs to be bathed in warm water in a warm room with no draughts. Babies do not maintain their temperature very well and need help to maintain it accordingly. Their temperature is maintained by a process called thermoregulation but normal temperature does not always equal a good environment. Babies may be maintaining their body temperature by using up their own energy stores and compromising their own natural defences. Sick babies' temperature regulation is impaired as it is already compromised.

There may be other signs that a baby has an infection, for example his or her muscle tone may not be good, the baby seems limp and inactive when awake. A well baby may look around and wriggle and grasp your finger if you place it across the palm of the baby's hand. The baby should also have a lusty cry and actively take his or her food on demand. In an unwell baby, the cry isn't as strong and she or he may not feed well. The latter is particularly true with babies who have jaundice as they become very sleepy and are uninterested in feeding. If you or the mother become concerned about a baby inform a midwife who can offer advice and any necessary treatment.

Nappies

New babies do pass urine, which can sometimes be masked by the amount of meconium passed. Meconium is the build up of waste products in the baby's gut during pregnancy. Baby girls, within the first few days of life, may have a small bleed into their nappies. This is perfectly normal, is called a 'pseudo-menstruation' and is caused by an influx of maternal hormones that have crossed the placenta and subsequently dropped in level. Parents should be reassured that this is perfectly normal with a simple explanation. If you or the mother should notice a pinky-orange substance in the nappy, inform the midwife who can provide advice and reassurance if necessary.

Babies' stools change colour over the first few days of life. They start with meconium, which is very dark green in colour and looks like tar. The amount initially passed can seem quite generous with new parents needing help, support and education on how to change a nappy. The stools then gradually change to a green colour. How the baby is fed will determine the colour. With bottle-fed babies, the colour becomes a mustardy yellow with 'seeds' in it. In contrast a breast-fed baby's stools are runny and khaki in colour.

Bathing and nappy changing

Help the new mother with bathing and show her how to change a nappy. Support new mums with this and perform a demonstration of either if required. Whilst in the clinical area you will be shown how to change nappies and bathe babies in line with your unit's policy. While bathing a baby (Fig. 14.1) it is important to keep the room warm and free of draughts as babies lose heat particularly quickly when they are wet.

Cord care

The umbilical cord is situated centrally in the abdomen. The cord was used for supplying the baby with nutrients from the placenta while the woman was pregnant. Once the baby has been born, the cord will have been clamped and cut by the midwife and over the next 7–10 days the cord will dry and then drop off. Many new mothers will worry that the cord, while it remains attached, is hurting the baby. However, it does not as there are no nerve endings in it.

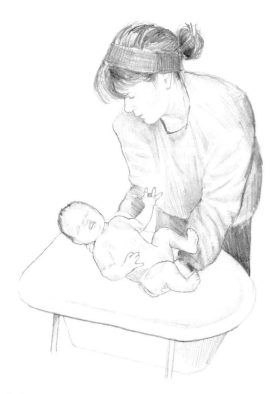

Fig. 14.1 Bathing baby.

It is important to keep the area of the cord clean and dry, as the cord is a potential source of infection. Cord care will be demonstrated to you in your clinical area. Certain powders were once used in the belief that they helped the cord dry up. These are no longer used as it was found that they did not speed up the process. Clean water and cotton wool can be used to keep the area clean. Once the area has been washed, ensure that it is dried well to help prevent any infection. If the base of the cord appears sticky, it may need cleaning but do inform a midwife. If you or the mother have any concerns regarding the cord area, speak to a midwife. This also includes any bleeding from the cord area. A baby needs to lose only a small amount of blood for this to be life-threatening.

Security

While babies are in hospital, they will have two labels placed on them to identify who they belong to. The labels need to remain in place while a baby is in hospital to prevent any mix-ups. If the labels are not present or you are not certain they are correct, inform the midwife who can action this immediately. Do not give the baby to someone you cannot identify.

Infant nutrition

A woman has a choice of how to feed her baby. She can either breast- or bottle-feed. Each unit has a policy on feeding babies. It is recognised that breast-feeding is better for a baby for a number of reasons, including that it is free, always on tap for the baby, contains the right nutrients at the right time for the baby and helps the baby's immune system. You must remember that not all women wish to breast-feed. When the woman has her baby, she may have already chosen to bottle-feed and she should be supported in her choice.

Breast-feeding

Although breast-feeding is natural, it is still a skill that needs to be learnt. In today's society, women may not have had an opportunity to learn from their family and friends about breast-feeding. It is therefore important that the midwife and health care professionals provide information to assist women to succeed in breast-feeding.

Once a baby has been born there is a drop in the level of a hormone called progesterone; this drop stimulates the release of another hormone called prolactin that stimulates the breasts to produce milk. After birth, the breasts produce colostrum. Colostrum is beneficial to the baby as it contains maternal antibodies that help build up undeveloped immune systems. At some point around day two to three, the woman's breasts may become engorged, firstly through venous engorgement (increase in blood flow to the breasts to adjust them for milk production), which is followed by milk engorgement. This can be very uncomfortable – you should reassure the mother of her normality, ensure that the baby is latching on correctly and encourage the woman to wear a supportive bra. In some cases cabbage leaves can be applied to help reduce the symptoms of engorgement. Engorgement may last a few days, with the breasts adjusting to the requirements the baby has placed on them. Did you know that, as the baby grows and continues breast-feeding, the breast-milk adapts to the needs of the growing baby?

The baby should, ideally, be put to the breast within half an hour of delivery: studies show that babies fed so quickly after birth breast-feed for longer during the postnatal period. This may be difficult, however, with women who have had a caesarean section. When a baby feeds, she or he should feed from one side during one feed and the other side at the next one, to feed for as long as possible. This is to enable the baby to get the full benefits of breast milk, which are fore milk and hind milk. Fore milk, the initial part of the milk that the baby receives when she or he starts a feed, is a sweeter watery form of milk that provides hydration for the baby. Hind milk, the second part of the milk, is the thicker milk which contains the nutrients and carbohydrates required for the baby's growth and development. Parents do not need to give their babies water as their fluid requirements are met by their mother's breast milk. Babies should be breast-fed on demand. This is called baby-led feeding, allowing the baby to feed for as long as required. You may need to provide help to ensure that the baby is correctly latched on and is in the right position.

Before putting the baby to the breast, help make the mother comfortable, as she may be in one position for quite some time. She can either sit up (Fig. 14.2) or lie down, as she wishes. When the baby latches on, the baby should not just take the nipple; the nipple and a good proportion of the area around the nipple, the areola, should be within the baby's mouth. This aids the expulsion of milk and also stimulates the breasts to produce more milk. When the baby has correctly latched on, you should see the baby's lower lip folded over, with the upper lip in a pout. As the baby sucks you should not see his/her cheeks being sucked in. You may also see the baby's ear move as he or she sucks and also the breast tissue moving. Mothers should not experience pain around the nipple area when they are breast-feeding. If this occurs, then the baby may not be latched on correctly, so gently take the baby off the breast and re-attach.

When the baby feeds, she or he is stimulating the breasts to produce more milk for the next feed, so the breasts supply according to the baby's demands. You may be asked by mothers about how much babies take when they breast-feed but it is difficult to measure the amount. Reassure accordingly. Breast-fed babies should not require 'topping-up'.

One of the common problems of breast-feeding is cracked nipples, which can be caused or exacerbated by poor latching during breast-feeding. There are two ways of helping to ease this. The first is to ensure that the baby, when feeding, is latched onto the breast correctly. You can also ease the discomfort by advising the woman to express a small amount of breast milk on to the affected area and then exposing this to the air: this can help ease the discomfort and aid with healing. Should the woman have cracked nipples, inform the midwife and tell her about any advice you have given.

Activity 14.4

Make a list of any common 'myths' about breast-feeding.

This list may include:

- Feeding a baby for 10 minutes on each side at each feed. This is no longer recommended.
- Colostrum being 'witch's milk'. There are some cultures that do not believe colostrum is of any benefit to the baby and would rather wait until it has passed.
- Babies should be put to the breast every four hours.
- Women with small breasts cannot make a sufficient amount of milk.
- 'Preparing' breasts before a feed. Breasts do this themselves.
- Breasts need cleaning prior to each feed – if a mother's hygiene is good, they don't.

Bottle-feeding

Do provide the same amount of support to a mother who wishes to bottle-feed. She may need help to learn how to feed a baby, for example how to hold the

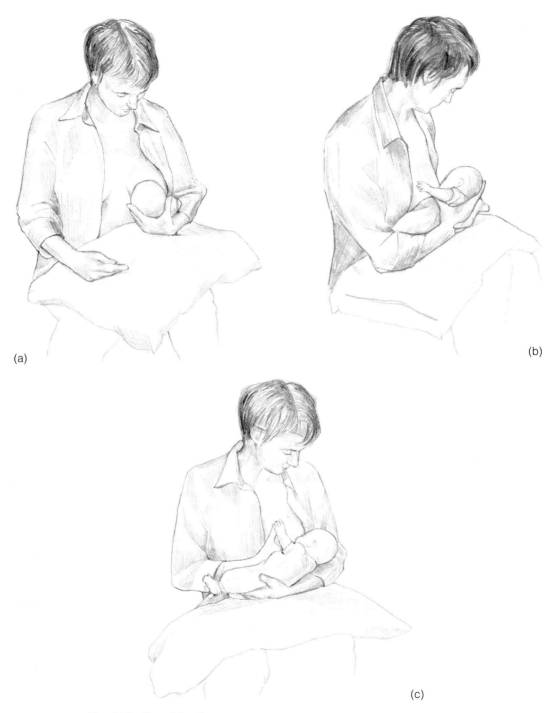

(a)

(b)

(c)

Fig. 14.2   Breast feeding.

baby and where to position the bottle. Once the baby has finished feeding from the bottle she or he may need *winding*. Depending upon the unit you work in, the woman may receive education on how to keep equipment clean and to make a feed. After a baby has finished feeding, document how the baby fed and how much was taken.

Activity 14.5

Think of the reasons that may influence a woman's choice of feeding. Examples may include peer pressure or previous experience.

You may encounter a situation when a mother is unable to feed her baby herself. If this is the case try to feed a baby in a suitable place, ideally with the mother. However, there may be occasions when a baby has been separated from his or her mother – for example, if the mother is too ill to feed her baby and requires specialised care in the labour ward.

Where the baby has problems taking food or does not appear to be feeding well, advice should be sought from the midwife or other appropriate professional without delay.

Feeding and interacting with the baby

Observe how the mother interacts with the baby, for example with feeding, holding and caring for the baby. Babies have certain senses developed quite early. They can recognise their mothers, through smell, voice and through seeing her. When a baby is in his or her mother's arms, the baby will watch her and seem transfixed by her. A new baby can see about 10 inches in front of them. This is the approximate distance between the mother's breast and face. A baby will also react if there are any sudden sounds and even at such a young age babies are now beginning to recognise his or her own mother's voice. When a new mother is learning to pick her new baby up, reassure her that the baby won't come to harm on being picked up. However, if you do notice that either parent of the baby is handling him or her too roughly or speaks negatively about the baby, you should immediately notify the midwife. The mother may be emotionally disturbed or the child might be at risk of abuse, with prompt action possibly helping the family to receive help needed in adjusting to having a new baby.

Mothers may need support in understanding their new baby's behaviour. Babies can cry for a number of reasons – hunger, needing a nappy change or just wanting a cuddle! A mother will soon learn her own baby's cry and what each cry means. Mothers may need to learn how to interact with their babies, for example, how to handle and talk to the baby. Some women may have to learn how to feed their babies; your job is to support them. You provide support and help to women, reiterating any advice given by the midwife.

The carer's role in supporting mothers in the first 10 postnatal days

An important aspect of your role in postnatal care is to reinforce professional advice by providing support and encouragement to women in the care of their babies. You must remember that your work is supervised by the midwife; any problems or difficulties experienced by the woman or baby should be seen by the midwife.

Documentation

Documentation of findings is important, not only because this makes sure that action is taken over any problem but also because there is a requirement for hospitals to keep records, which must be held for at least 25 years from the last entry. They are a legal entity and can be used in a court of law as evidence on the implementation of an individual's care. Therefore, accurate documentation of each individual is required.

Summary

Your role is to assist women in looking after themselves and their babies, as usually after the first day the main carer of a new baby is his or her mother. Different women will have different requirements – for example, a mother who has already had a child will have some knowledge of baby care.

The six weeks following the birth, the puerperium, is a time of great physiological and psychological change. The main professional in this time-frame is the midwife, who provides the initial care, support and education that a woman may need in the days following her baby's birth. During this time, you also support the mother by providing information and reiterating the advice given by a midwife in the course of her duty.

Your role in caring for mothers and babies postnatally is to assist the midwife. You will be working under her supervision and guidance at all times with all your help being greatly appreciated.

References

1. United Kingdom Central Council for Nursing, Midwifery and Health Visiting (1998) *The Midwives' Rules and Code of Professional Conduct*. UKCC, London.
2. Niven (1995) *Psychological Care for New Families*, 3rd edition. Blackwell, Oxford, p. 252.

Further reading

Collins S. and Powell J. Postnatal depression. Available at www.netdoctor.co.uk/health_advice/facts/depressionpostnatal.htm (accessed 10 September 2002).

Eastman A. (2000) The mother-baby dance: positioning and latch-on. *Leaven* p. 63–68.

Henderson C. and Jones K. (1997) *Essential Midwifery*. CV Mosby, St Louis. p. 229–284.

Page L.A. (2000) *The New Midwifery*. Churchill Livingstone, Edinburgh, p. 210, 340–348.

Rowe-Murray, H.J. and Fisher J.R.W. (2002) Baby friendly hospital practices: caesarean section is a persistent barrier to early initiation of breast-feeding. *Birth* **2** (2), 124–130.

Chapter 15

Caring for children and their families

Lisa S. Whiting

Overview

In this chapter we will consider the principles of care for the child and family. Attention will be paid to the effects of hospitalisation, the role of the family, the importance of play and the maintenance of a safe environment. Psychological care will be considered throughout, but specific physical care will not be included since it is beyond the scope of this chapter.

Key words: Child; family; separation; partnership; play; communication; safety; child abuse

Effects of hospitalisation

As a child you may have been in hospital and you may have memories of how it felt. Clearly, hospitalisation may impact upon children and their families in a variety of ways. This section of the chapter will focus upon the effects of hospitalisation and how they relate to children. One of the main issues is *separation* of the child from family, friends, toys and the home environment. As carers, it is important to understand the possible effects of separation and to work with the child and family to minimise these. John Bowlby, an eminent psychiatrist who specialised in child psychology, believed that[1]:

> the infant and young child should experience a warm, intimate, and continuous relationship with his mother (or permanent mother substitute) in which both find satisfaction and enjoyment.

When Bowlby was conducting his work, it was common practice for children in hospital to be separated from their families and for visiting to be very restricted, for example once, a week and parents only. This was thought to be advantageous as the children became distressed when their parents left. Today, families are encouraged to spend as much time as possible with their child.

Despite this, parental separation does still occur for a variety of reasons (for example, many parents work and are having to 'juggle' family and job commitments). In view of this, it is essential that we understand how separation may affect a child.

Research by James Robertson, originally a social worker, identified stages of adjustment that young children exhibit when separated from their families[2]. He suggested that the child between six months and four years of age is particularly vulnerable to the effects of separation and hospitalisation:

> If at this crucial stage in his development, when he has such a possessive and passionate need for his mother, and he is blindly trustful of his parents, he is admitted alone to hospital, he experiences a serious failure of that environment of love and security hitherto provided by his family and which we know to be a necessary experience if he is to be a loving, secure and trustful person in later life.

The effects of separation, as identified by Robertson, are given below. Such reactions may be seen even when the period of separation is brief.

Protest

- The child is grief-stricken, calling constantly for the parent(s). As the young child lives in the present he may feel deserted by parents.
- The child is likely to reject the hospital carer and may become openly hostile.

Despair

- The child sinks into apparent depression, becoming quiet, apathetic and withdrawn, mourning for the lost parent(s).
- The child may adopt self-comforting behaviours, such as thumb sucking, and may regress developmentally, for example in potty training, play activities or language.
- The child may exhibit behavioural difficulties and sleep problems.
- When parents visit, the child may become upset.

Denial

- The child no longer appears depressed and shows interest in the immediate surroundings.
- The child may now repress all feelings for the parent(s).
- If the child has a prolonged hospital stay, he may settle into the routine and way of life. This may lead to long-term emotional disturbances.
- The child might also become the 'pet' of carers, receiving 'special' attention and care.

Although it is generally agreed that young children are most susceptible to the effects of separation and hospitalisation, children of any age who require repeated admissions, or whose condition necessitates a single protracted period in hospital, are also at risk[3,4].

Activity 15.1

Take some time to observe children in your work area. Do any of them exhibit any signs of the behaviours identified above?

Many other problems are associated with the hospitalisation of children. Take time to consider other effects on the child, the parents, brothers and/or sisters (siblings) and make a list of points.

Your list may include all or some of the following discussed below.

Effects on the child

- Disruption of home routine, particularly important for the very young child.
- The child may become very confused, fearful of being hurt, and may then revert to baby-like behaviour which is known as regression.
- School-work may be neglected.
- The child may not sleep properly.

Effects on the parents

- Parents may feel that they need to be in two places at once, i.e. with their child and at home with the rest of the family.
- Parents may have feelings of guilt, particularly if their child has been admitted to hospital as a result of a preventable accident.
- Clearly anxiety for the welfare of their child will be significant for the majority of parents.
- Financial problems may arise, e.g. loss of earnings or extra expenses incurred for travelling.
- Parents may become physically and emotionally exhausted.
- Bonding between baby and parents may be reduced.
- The whole family may be thrown into turmoil and 'crisis' which may compound the feelings of parents.

Effects on the siblings

Siblings may express a number of feelings and it is important to remember that the sibling may also be experiencing separation if a parent is resident with a hospitalised child. Morrison found that the sibling may exhibit signs of nervousness and sadness and sleep and school problems[5]. Other feelings could include:

- Guilt that they may somehow have caused the child's illness
- Resentment and jealousy that they are receiving less attention than the sick child
- Anger that they are not kept informed of the child's illness, or invited to participate in the care
- Fear and anxiety about their sibling and how well they are recovering

- Loneliness – even siblings who don't appear to have strong bonds may miss each other desperately. This may be amplified if the well child is being cared for by friends and relatives with whom they are not very familiar.

In recognition of these potentially damaging effects upon the child and family, the Platt Report[6], as long ago as 1959, recommended that the child should not be admitted to hospital if it can possibly be avoided. However, if it is necessary, the degree to which a young child may become disturbed because of separation depends on a number of factors. These are identified below:

- The child's age and stage of development.
- The nature of the child/parent relationship.
- The seriousness of the child's illness.
- The frequency of previous separations. The child who has been in hospital on a number of previous occasions may appear to adapt to the next admission more easily than the child who has never been away from parents or stayed away from home overnight. It is important to remember, however, that appearances may be deceptive. The quiet, composed child may be experiencing inner turmoil.
- The preparation that the child received prior to admission. It may be well nigh impossible to prepare the child admitted as a result of sudden illness or accident. However, for the child whose admission is planned, both physical and psychological preparation can be made. This preparation will be discussed later.
- The role of parents while the child is in hospital. Continuous contact with parents during the child's stay is vital. If one parent can be resident, this will help to maintain security and stability for the child.
- The amount of sensory stimulation that the child receives. The provision of appropriate play materials, suitable for the child's developmental age, is essential.
- The parents' response to changed events and routine. Children are particularly receptive to the way their parents react, and this can have an important influence on the experience of being in hospital.
- The support and advice which is available to the child and family.

These factors affect the child while in hospital, but it is equally important to remember that they will also affect the child's behaviour after they return home.

Easing the effects of separation

Activity 15.2

We have identified some of the effects of hospitalisation for both the child and the family. It is becoming clear that they need to be minimised as far as possible. Either by yourself or with a group of colleagues, make a list of some actions that could be taken to reduce some of these problems.

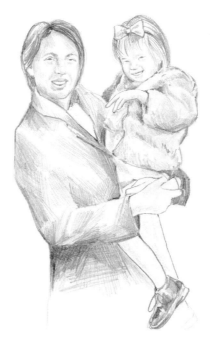

Fig. 15.1   Mother and child enjoy time together.

Some of your solutions may include the following:

- Encourage parent(s) to spend as much time as possible with their child (Fig. 15.1). There can be no doubt that illness makes the child more dependent and increases the need for close contact with the family. Where possible the parent(s) should be offered the opportunity to be resident with their child, but pressure should not be applied. If it is not possible, why not suggest that the parent leaves an item of soft clothing with the child, this will provide a sense of security and comfort.
- Encourage the whole family to participate in the child's care, provided they are willing and happy to do so and have received any necessary instruction.
- As carers we can help by staying with the child when the parent(s) are not visiting. The use of diversional play can be very valuable, as can cuddling and comforting the child.
- Preserve, as far as possible, the child's home routine, such as bedtime, bath time, story time.
- Ask parents to bring the child's usual and favourite toys/comforters. Parents may feel embarrassed that their 4- or 5-year-old still has a dummy; reassurance needs to be given that this is not the time to remove the comforter; in fact it may be of more help than usual.
- Encourage siblings to visit and be involved in care. Adolescents may particularly value seeing their friends and peers.
- Share information with the whole family about the child's care and management on a regular basis. Questions should be answered and information

expressed in understandable terms. Strategies employed to reduce parental anxiety can be expected to have both direct and indirect benefits for the child.

- Psychological preparation of the child for procedures, for example the taking of blood, administration of drugs or an operation, is clearly of paramount importance if distress is to be limited. Consider the child's age and development stage when explaining what will happen and think about using resources like books and toys which may assist you. In addition, other personnel, such as the play therapist, may have a valuable role in these circumstances – do draw on the available expertise. If you should have any concerns about the child's level of anxiety, ensure that you inform the relevant member of the multi-disciplinary team.
- Keep the number of carers involved in the child's care to a minimum to avoid the confusion created by too many strangers and, more importantly, to give the family ample opportunity to build and preserve relationships.
- Take time to listen and talk with the child. This is clearly important for all children, but is particularly significant for the adolescent. Burr suggested that little consideration is given to this age group and the facilitation of their independent stay in hospital[7].

It is clear that a period in hospital can have a profound effect upon the psychological welfare of the child. It is therefore our responsibility to attempt to minimise problems and to work towards returning the child to their home environment and family as soon as possible. However, it is essential to remember that a visit to hospital can be a positive experience, for example, allowing opportunities for children and their families to meet others with similar problems, providing security, helping the development of social interaction, and of course, facilitating the return to an optimum state of health.

Care in partnership with the family

The involvement of the family in the care of the child in hospital has already been mentioned. As this is such an important feature, we will now explore it in more detail. White and Woollett suggest that 'For most people the family is by far the most significant institution in terms of the impact it has on the quality of their daily life and experience'[8].

A great many authors, in particular sociologists, have attempted to define the term family. Murdock describes the family as being a social group who live together, the group including male and female adults, two of whom maintain a socially approved sexual relationship and have one or more children[9]. This definition perhaps reflects the lifestyles which were prevalent at the time of writing. More recently, Bond and Bond offer the view that the family is a universal institution taking many forms within one culture and between different cultures[10]. This stance is echoed by Bruce and Meggitt who suggest that there is no such thing as a standard family, each one being different and individually embracing a range of cultures and perspectives[11].

Almost all of us have an in-depth knowledge and closeness with at least one family, and this may influence our personal opinions of what constitutes a family. You may have noticed how your own particular family differs in its organisational structure from those of your friends. In the UK, many families have a nuclear structure (parents and children live separately from other relatives); others have an extended structure (a range of relatives live together in a close-knit community). In some families the mother is the central figure – sociologists call this the matriarchal family, while other families are father-centred and this is the patriarchal family. Some families are neither mother nor father centred and some are single-parent families.

Activity 15.3

Consider families which you know and try to identify the description given above which best fits them.

The family has become idealised within many cultures, being seen as valuable, good and worthwhile. However, it is evident that it has evolved and developed over the generations to meet our diverse needs. Changes in society influence family life and values, and the changes today are many, rapid, varied and far reaching. Demographic trends indicate that people tend to have fewer children than they did 50 years ago. Contraception is widely available and termination of pregnancy is legal. Families are subjected to a number of social pressures, such as maintaining a high standard of living and, as a result, many women return to work after the birth of their children in order to contribute to the family's finances.

Alterations in lifestyle also include unemployment; more adults choosing to cohabit rather than marry; increasing divorce rates and re-marriages leading to mixings of partners and their children. Finally, growing numbers of different ethnic groups are represented in our society, all of whom have differing values and cultures.

A fair conclusion would be that the image of Mr and Mrs Average with their two children – the family – may be difficult to find! Despite the complexity of family structures and the difficulties which they may present, there is overwhelming evidence to suggest that families are extremely important to children[12–14]. It is for this reason that the acceptance and reasonable understanding of different family structures and cultures is vital if we, as carers, are to work in partnership with *the whole family.*

Activity 15.4

From your experience, make a list of the different family structures you have encountered as part of your work.

Your list may be very extensive. Here are some possibilities:

- Two parents and their children, all from the same cultural background.
- Two parents and their children, parents from different cultural backgrounds.
- Parents who have adopted children from the same or a different cultural background.
- Families with their own children and others who are fostered.
- Parents who have conceived children by assisted means, such as egg or sperm donation, in vitro fertilisation, surrogacy.
- Two lesbians or homosexuals who have children (for example from previous marriages, fostering, adoption or assisted means).
- A one-parent family, as a result of:
  −divorce/separation
  −death of one partner
  −single (relationship with partner never fully established).

The nature of the family structure will, naturally, influence the beliefs, attitudes and values of its members. It is essential that we respect these, however, different they are from our own, and appreciate their importance.

Family reactions to a child's illness and hospitalisation

The Department of Health estimated that there are 11 000 000 children in England. Of these, approximately 1 683 000 (under the age of 15 years) had a hospital contact in the 12 months from 1 April to 31 March 1998[15,16]. To many families this event is the cause of great stress. For us, the carers, it is sometimes difficult to appreciate the anxiety parents experience. This may be particularly so if the child has been admitted for what seems to be a relatively minor treatment. However, it seems that parents' reactions and the degree of stress experienced vary little regardless of the child's diagnosis or the severity of the illness. The child is precious beyond measure to parents and no illness or treatment is small or unimportant. If the child is very sick the parents' reactions become more intense and persistent.

Activity 15.5

Make a note of how you think parents may react to their child's illness and hospitalisation.

You may have identified some of the following emotions:

- Disbelief: Especially if the illness is sudden.
- Guilt: The parent(s) may search for self-blame. They may ask 'Why is our child ill? Was it something we did?'
- Anger: Parents may vent angry feelings towards those caring for their child.
- Fear/anxiety may be directly related to the child's illness, or to the investigations/treatment to be carried out.

- Frustration can arise because the parent is given insufficient information about the child's illness and they may not understand what they are expected to do while their child is in hospital.
- Depression sometimes occurs while the child is in hospital, but can also cause problems following discharge. Parents may comment that they feel mentally and physically exhausted once the child is home. Their feelings may also be due to the child's long-term prognosis, any negative effects induced by the hospital stay and financial problems that may have arisen as a result.

Encouraging the family to become involved in the child's care

The family, and in particular the parents, may see the child's hospital stay as a very traumatic experience. Some of these feelings can be alleviated by encouraging them to be involved in the child's care.

When referring to family participation we think primarily of parents, but any member who plays a significant role in the child's upbringing may be involved. Encouraging siblings to participate helps to deal with some of the negative reactions which we described earlier, and also helps to maintain the family unit. *Partnership with the family* should be the focus of all the care given to the child in hospital.

Activity 15.6

Make some notes about how you think you could encourage the family to participate in their child's care.

Your notes may include some of the points discussed below.

Encouragement

A parent may become extremely distressed when someone else is caring for their child. Encouraging one or more family members to spend as much time as possible with the child provides opportunity for them to be involved in planning and giving care and possibly hastens the child's recovery. Families may carry out the child's washing and feeding or wish to be involved in areas of care new to them. There is no reason why the family should not take over responsibility for any aspect of their child's care provided they are happy to do so and they receive appropriate preparation and support. However, not all families feel comfortable taking this kind of responsibility so it is important not to pressurise them.

Recognising parents as experts

Some families will be highly skilled in caring for their child, particularly if the child has a chronic disease. All parents are able to offer valuable advice and information about their child's normal home routine and lifestyle.

Providing support

This involves willingness to listen and respond to the family's concerns and anxieties. This may help parents to accept their own feelings towards their sick child. Support could also be more practical help, such as offering to sit and cuddle the child while the parent goes for a cup of tea.

Offering advice

This may be advice about how to carry out any aspect of the child's care. Alternatively, it may be suggesting to other relatives how they might help, for example caring for other children at home or doing household chores, so that parents are relieved of some of these burdens.

Accepting family cultural, socio-economic and ethnic values

The parents may wish to introduce others they regard as important to their child's care, for example a representative of their religious faith or a practitioner of a complementary therapy such as massage. Medical advice may need to be sought for the latter.

Providing advice and information

If the parents are fully aware of the child's illness and the planned management, much anxiety is relieved. The sick child, if old enough, and other family members may need to be involved in these discussions. Explanations of how siblings may react to the child's hospitalisation will help parents to appreciate the need to involve them in the care.

Caring team

The child should be cared for by as few people as possible to give continuity of care and to give the parents the opportunity to build relationships, confidence and a sense of control, making them feel part of the team.

The multi-disciplinary team

Other personnel may be involved in the child's care, such as doctors, social workers, speech therapists, physiotherapists, and it is important that a team approach is employed and that individuals do not operate in isolation.

To summarise, the following three points encapsulate the discussion:

- Ask the family for which aspects of care they would like to take responsibility.
- Build the family's confidence by giving reassurance and information.
- Give the family support and encouragement when they are giving care.

Role of the carer

Now a word about carers. Although when caring for children, the client/carer relationship is extended owing to the presence of the family, the responsibility for care still lies with the registered practitioner whom you are assisting. Initially you may find it stressful working closely with the family, and may even feel that you are under their scrutiny – indeed those of you who are parents may readily appreciate the family's viewpoint in this matter. However, this is something that you will become used to in time – remember caring for the child in partnership with the family can greatly enhance the child's recovery.

One area of your role which is growing in importance is that of health promotion. Since this also involves working with both the child and family, it would seem that this is an opportune point to briefly consider the areas of health promotion in which you could participate. You may already be familiar with the term 'health promotion' – it has been receiving increased attention during the past decade, particularly in respect of children. The World Health Organization has defined health promotion as 'The process of enabling people to increase control over, and to improve, their health'[17]. Bunton and Macdonald provide a broad description by stating that health promotion 'represents at the very simplest level . . . a strategy for promoting, in some positive way, the health of whole populations'[18].

It is clear from these views that health promotion may embrace all aspects of your role – it could be argued that everything you are doing is promoting health in some way. We are sure that you will be asked for advice in relation to an array of health issues pertaining to children and their families, perhaps including areas such as feeding, accident prevention or play. You will feel comfortable addressing some points, but others will require referral to other members of staff. In addition to your advisory role, you may be provided with the opportunity to participate in a range of other health promotion activities as a member of the health care team. Examples could include involvement in:

- Pre-hospital admission programmes
- Visits to schools
- Preparing information for parent education notice boards

We feel that this is an important aspect of your role. Health promotion necessitates that children, their families and *all* members of the multi-disciplinary care team work together to enable each child to fulfil their potential and to reach their optimal level of health.

The child and play

Play is an essential part of every child's life and vital to the process of human development[18]. Bruce and Meggitt go further by stating that play 'brings together the ideas, feelings, relationships and physical life of the child'[11].

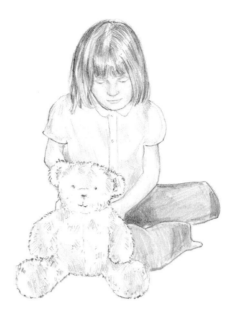

Fig. 15.2   Child at play.

As the child's life needs to progress as normally as possible, we will examine the stages and types of play, the provision of play for the child in hospital and how play can be used as a part of care (Fig. 15.2).

Stages of play

Play has many functions and purposes. Individual children play in different ways – some quietly, others noisily and actively. Despite these apparent differences, children generally adopt styles of play according to their age.

- Solitary play: is adopted by young children up to approximately 2 years of age. They prefer to play alone, although like to have a parent or familiar person nearby. At this stage repetition is important – you may have seen a young child deriving great amusement from repeatedly throwing a toy or teddy out of the cot.
- Parallel play: Children between 3 and 4 years of age enjoy playing alongside each other. They may briefly interact, perhaps to show one another an interesting object, but each child continues to play independently for most of the time.
- Social play: At approximately 4 years of age the child has usually begun to play with others in small groups of perhaps two, three or four. At this stage children are learning to share and interact with others but they will still use solitary and parallel play.

Types of play

There are many types of play and you will see that these are described in a variety of ways by different authors. However, whatever terminology is used, all play aims to develop particular skills in the child. Ideally, the child should have the opportunity to participate in a range of play throughout childhood. Examples include:

- Rough and tumble play
- Exploratory play
- Constructive play
- Manipulative play
- Make-believe play
- Role play
- Social play
- Problem-solving play
- Games with rules
- Hobbies

In addition, you may hear the term 'therapeutic play' which is facilitated by those who have undertaken specialised professional training to help children who are experiencing emotional pain to explore their feelings.

The carer's role in relation to play

Children need adults to help them to play and to provide them with suitable play materials. It is particularly important to remember that children who are sick, unhappy or disabled may experience difficulties playing and will require your support even more. However, at the same time, your style should not be too directive, allowing the child to use their imagination. Sometimes one can feel lost and not know *how to play* with children. The following suggestions may help:

- Make yourself comfortable and sit at the child's level.
- Introduce the child to others so that they have the opportunity to play together. This is particularly important for those who are 4 years of age and over.
- Give praise and encouragement to the child if they accomplish something well, for example a 2-year-old completing a simple jigsaw puzzle. At the same time, try not to reinforce negative behaviour such as a child hitting another with a toy hammer! The most suitable action is to tell the child kindly but firmly that this is wrong. It may be necessary to physically separate the children and divert their attentions with other games.
- Join in with the child's play, for example board games, role play, hospital play.
- Ensure that all children in your care have equal opportunities to participate in play, irrespective of age, culture or disability.
- At all times consider the safety of children while they are at play. This includes factors such as adequate supervision and the provision of toys that conform to British and European standards.
- Respect the family's cultural, religious and social beliefs in the course of play.

Activity 15.7

What play facilities/materials would you suggest as appropriate for children of the following ages? Give two examples for each age group:

Birth to 6 months
6 months to 1 year
1–2 years
2–3 years
3–5 years
5–7 years
8–12 years
12 years onwards

Here are a few suggestions to complete Activity 15.7.

Birth to 6 months

Babies of this age like colourful objects they can watch and listen to such as mobiles, rattles, mirrors and soft cuddly toys. They also enjoy activities such as finger play.

6 months to 1 year

These babies will be becoming more inquisitive and will need toys that give them the opportunity to develop skills. Examples include activity centres and mats, building bricks, toy telephone, and they usually love playing in the bath with buckets or squeezy toys.

1–2 years

The child at this age has begun to explore – many are very mobile. Suitable play materials include push-along toys, posting boxes, toys that they sit and ride on, simple jigsaws and stacking toys.

2–3 years

Children of this age particularly enjoy make-believe play and dressing up. Appropriate play materials would include old clothes, dolls, domestic equipment like saucepans, tea sets, large nuts and bolts, sandpit with bucket and spade. At the same time the child has developed more advanced motor movement, so objects like large beads to make a necklace, paints and brushes, climbing frames and swings will also be popular.

3–5 years

This group is acquiring new skills very rapidly. They enjoy construction toys, larger jigsaws, cutting-out (with blunt scissors), making collages, playing doctors and nurses, play-dough, finger-painting, Wendy houses.

5–7 years

Children of this age like to make things, so simple embroidery, cookery, basic woodwork, for example, may be suitable. They also enjoy more active games like football and skipping.

8–12 years

More complex toys that require a certain amount of skill can now be introduced, such as computer and board games. They may also, by now, have a number of hobbies: cooking, swimming, horse riding to name a few.

12 years onwards

This age group is more interested in pursuing individual interests and hobbies, so it is important to identify what these are. Most common examples include listening to music, talking with friends, sport activities and computer games.

The above are just a few ideas that you may find helpful in your work. Most importantly, it is essential to identify the child's individual interests and seek to accommodate these.

Play for the child in hospital

Play for the hospitalised child 'is one of the few elements of normal life in an abnormal situation'[20]. It should be available to all children, in whichever department they are being cared for, including casualty and out-patient departments, because it fulfils so many vital functions.

Play promotes continuation of growth and development and helps to minimise regression. It can help the child to deal with the stress of the situation and gives the child the opportunity to express feelings and emotions. By reducing anxiety it can speed recovery and therefore shorten the hospital stay.

It can form excellent diversional therapy, occupy the child and prevent or relieve boredom. Play can enable children to relate to staff, and prepare them for their hospital admission and for medical procedures such as blood tests, scans and surgery. It may also reduce parental anxiety as it allows the family to participate in some of the child's normal activities. We have already identified that when children are ill and in hospital some aspects of their development may regress. For this same reason, children may choose to play with toys which make them feel comfortable and secure, but are more suited to a younger age group – this does not need to be discouraged. In addition, concentration span and interest in a particular toy may be limited, so a variety of play materials should be available. Observation of the child at play is important and may give the first indication of emotional upset or regression. As carers we may be the first to notice these changes.

All children in hospital should be encouraged to play in some form, however sick or disabled they may be. However, it is important to recognise that the illness or necessary treatment may limit both the child's capacity for and interest in play.

Using play to prepare a child for medical procedures

Play can also be used to help prepare children for medical procedures such as an operation. Your work area may have a hospital corner which has a stock of bandages, theatre masks and hats, stethoscopes and books. Children may ask you to participate in their hospital play, for example to be a client or to help bandage teddy's arm.

Let us consider an example of using play towards a child's treatment.

Activity 15.8

Samir is 5 years old and has been admitted to hospital for removal of his adenoids and tonsils. Make some notes to cover how you think play therapy could be used to help prepare him for his operation.

Your notes may include some of the following points:

- Identify Samir's present level of knowledge. What does he know about his forthcoming operation? Has he been in hospital before? What have his parents told him and what toys or books have they used to help prepare him for the admission and the surgery?
- Establish how Samir feels about his operation. Is he frightened? Or is he calm and relaxed? This will influence the amount and intensity of preparation required.

When these questions have been answered, Samir's knowledge can be built upon during the pre-operative period. A number of methods can be used to help prepare Samir for this operation.

- Books telling stories about children coming into hospital can be read to him and he may enjoy looking at the pictures. (Suitable books are listed at the end of this chapter.) Booklets and photograph albums may be available to explain procedures and care for children in your specific area.
- Some clinical areas have videos depicting children going to theatre for particular operations. (Examples of appropriate videos which may be purchased are also provided at the end of the chapter). If available, these may prove very useful, along with someone available to answer Samir's and his parents' questions.
- Samir's favourite toys may be included in the preparation, particularly if they are going to accompany him to theatre. Samir may like teddy to be a client too and so the opportunity exists for Samir to see and hear what will happen when he is prepared for operation by demonstrating and explaining using teddy. Then when Samir goes for his operation teddy can go too.

Clear, truthful explanations appropriate to Samir's level of understanding are essential. It is particularly important to explain to Samir when he will go home and to discuss any unpleasant side-effects that he may experience afterwards, such as a sore throat. To be truthful is to preserve the child's trust. You may find that both child and parent(s) need the information repeated a number of times to give them a chance to absorb what is being said.

Family members should be involved in all aspects of the child's preparation. You may find that little preparation is required for some children going to theatre, for others more time and a combination of techniques may be appropriate. Clearly these points could easily be adapted to help prepare children who are to undergo other medical procedures and treatments, such as insertion of intravenous infusions, scans, x-rays, physiotherapy and speech therapy. The planned psychological preparation of a child is not always fully successful, but it does help allay the anxiety in many children and their parents.

Other functions of play

Play has a number of other functions, for example children may use it to express their emotions. A child who has suffered abuse may use a doll or teddy to role play experiences; a teenager who is going through an emotional crisis may express feelings in drawings or poetry. For this reason, it is vital that we observe and listen to children at play and take their views and actions seriously. If you are concerned or worried about the significance of a child's play, do not hesitate to convey this to a senior member of staff.

Finally, we can also incorporate play into a child's care and management. For example, Chloe is 5 years old and has cystic fibrosis and needs to practise deep breathing exercises to help improve her lung function. This could be made more fun by encouraging her to blow bubbles. Likewise, Jake has cerebral palsy and the fine movement and co-ordination of his fingers are poor, so the use of jigsaw puzzles may prove beneficial. Or, 1-year-old Olivia requires physiotherapy for her legs; toys may divert her attention while she is undergoing her exercises.

We see that play is vital to the growth and development of the child, and that it has a particularly significant role for those in hospital. It is our responsibility to ensure that all children in our care have the opportunity to experience a variety of play activities appropriate to their individual needs.

Maintaining a safe environment for the child in hospital

The last part of this chapter is devoted to issues concerned with child safety. Unfortunately, accidents create the need for a considerable number of child admissions to hospital and, more sadly, accidents do happen in hospital. Although all references to safety throughout this book apply equally to the care of children, as a conclusion we will explore important safety aspects which are specific to them.

Accidents

Accidents are *the* major health problem for children under the age of 14 years. Children's accidents resulted in 423 deaths, and approximately 2280000 casualty department attendances in the UK in 1999[21]. Thus, accidents are clearly a significant cause of distress for both the child and family. You will probably be involved in the care of children who have been admitted to hospital as a result of an accident – perhaps due to a fall, a scald or the inhalation or swallowing of a foreign body.

A significant number of accidents (over a million each year) occur in the home environment[21]. However, it could be argued that there are more potential hazards in hospital than in the child's home, so extra precautions need to be taken to ensure that the environment is as safe as possible.

Environmental hazards in the hospital

We will now consider some of the environmental hazards. It is important to remember that hospital is a strange environment for the child and family, so this alone may increase the risk of accidents.

Activity 15.9

Look around your clinical area and make a list of the environmental hazards that could cause accidental injury to a child.

No doubt you will have many ideas, here are a few suggestions:

- Hot drinks left on bedside lockers.
- Toys: a toddler or child may inhale or swallow small parts of toys and children may trip over toys.
- Equipment such as intravenous infusion pumps: a young child may walk into the pump and its stand; a child may play with the plug/plug socket/buttons of the infusion pump.
- Sharp objects not correctly disposed of.
- Unattended drug trolley.
- Ward door left open: all clinical areas should have child safety doors and a security system. It is essential to ensure that these are fully operational and used correctly at all times.
- Spillages on floors causing a parent or child to slip.
- Uniform accessories of carers, such as badges with sharp edges (these may be harmful when cuddling a child), or scissors that can easily be pulled from your pocket.
- Radiators could be a potential cause of burns; all should have radiator guards.
- Windows are particularly hazardous if your clinical area is not on the ground floor; window guards and child safety locks are essential.
- Hot water taps.

Safety precautions in hospital

Apart from environmental factors, accidents can occur if hospital procedures or protocols are not strictly adhered to. No doubt we have all read newspaper articles about clients who have had the wrong surgery or drugs. Young children are perhaps even more at risk, since their verbal communication skills are limited. The following are examples of how we can all work towards ensuring that the child's planned care and management is carried out safely and uneventfully.

Name band

All children should have a name band on their wrist or ankle, correctly completed with name, date of birth and hospital number. If it needs to be removed, another should replace it immediately.

General anaesthesia

All necessary documentation must be completed, and all hospital policies carefully followed for all children who are to undergo a general anaesthetic.

Protection from infection

The hospital environment contains a variety of viruses and bacteria and, wherever possible, children need to be protected from these. Those particularly at risk are the sick, children whose natural defence systems are not efficient and the young baby whose own immune system is immature, and who has yet to develop protective antibodies. Handwashing must be thorough and other necessary precautions, such as nursing the child in a cubicle, carried out.

In particular, those children who are admitted to hospital as a result of an infectious disease need to be nursed in a cubicle, with both carers and family adhering to the infection control policy. This should limit the spread of infection. This subject is covered in greater detail in Chapter 9.

Drug administration

Hospital policy must be carefully followed. The child's name band should always be checked prior to giving medicines, and no drug should ever be left unattended on tables or lockers.

Provision of sterile and correctly diluted infant feeds

The feeds, feeding equipment and dummies for babies up to 1 year of age should be sterile. This may be facilitated by the use of ready prepared bottle formula milks. Any remaining milk should be disposed of immediately after feeding since it is an ideal medium for the growth of bacteria.

Positioning, moving and handling of children

You should be provided with the opportunity to attend study sessions relating to the positioning, moving and handling of children. This is an integral aspect of care which may not only facilitate recovery and return to optimal health, but also prevent any deterioration or other further problems developing. In addition, it will help you to protect yourself from unnecessary injury.

Fire

All staff working within a hospital must be aware of the fire regulations and procedures.

Policies relating to all of the above points are available in your own clinical areas and you should be familiar with them. Safety is an essential component of a child's care and it is our responsibility as carers to maintain protective measures throughout the child's stay.

Protecting the child from abuse

It is impossible to know the precise incidence of child abuse; however, of the 11 000 000 children who reside in England, it is estimated that between 300 000 and 400 000 are known to Social Services and 32 000 have their names on a child protection register at any one time[15]. This is probably the tip of the iceberg and thousands more children may suffer long-term psychological problems as a result of ill treatment. There is no doubt that public concern has increased in relation to child protection and this has been reflected in legislation, the Children Act being of significant importance[22].

As you will be involved in the direct care of children – bathing, washing, talking and listening to them – it may be you who is in a position to identify either potential or actual child abuse and consequently maintain the child's safety.

What is child abuse?

There are four identified forms of abuse:

- Physical abuse
- Neglect
- Sexual abuse
- Emotional abuse

The Department of Health has developed clear and precise definitions relating to each area[23], these are presented below to allow you to fully appreciate the possible diversity of child abuse.

Physical abuse

Physical abuse may involve hitting, shaking, throwing, poisoning, burning or scalding, drowning, suffocating, or otherwise causing physical harm to a child. Physical harm may also be caused when a parent or carer feigns the symptoms of, or deliberately causes ill health to a child whom they are looking after. This situation is commonly described using terms such as factitious illness by proxy or Munchausen syndrome by proxy.

(Department of Health, 1999[23])

Neglect

Neglect is the persistent failure to meet a child's basic physical and/or psychological needs, likely to result in the serious impairment of the child's health or development. It may involve a parent or carer failing to provide adequate food, shelter and clothing, failing to protect a child from physical harm or danger, or the failure to ensure access to appropriate medical care or treatment. It may also include neglect of, or unresponsiveness to, a child's basic emotional needs.

(Department of Health, 1999[23])

Sexual abuse

Sexual abuse involves forcing or enticing a child or young person to take part in sexual activities, whether or not the child is aware of what is happening. The activities may involve physical contact, including penetrative (rape or buggery) or non-penetrative acts. They may include non-contact activities, such as involving children in looking at, or the production of, pornographic material or watching sexual activities, or encouraging children to behave in sexually inappropriate ways.

(Department of Health, 1999[23])

Emotional abuse

Emotional abuse is the persistent emotional ill-treatment of a child such as to cause severe and persistent adverse effects on the child's emotional development. It may involve conveying to children that they are worthless or unloved, inadequate, or valued only insofar as they meet the needs of another person. It may feature age or developmentally inappropriate expectations being imposed upon children. It may involve causing children to feel frightened or in danger, or the exploitation or corruption of children. Some level of emotional abuse is involved in all types of ill-treatment of a child, though it may occur alone.

(Department of Health, 1999[23])

Detecting child abuse

Abuse can have profound effects upon a child and, sadly, it is not as rare and unusual as is sometimes thought. Child abuse can affect *any* family, so prevention, early detection and supportive help and advice are crucial to the well-being of the child and family. The most severe cases of child abuse are usually not difficult to identify, but not all incidents are clear-cut.

Activity 15.10

Consider the following examples. Would you think them to be child abuse?

- An 8-year-old boy who is forced, each evening, by his parents, to do two hours of Maths or English homework
- A 6-year-old girl who always has her bedtime bath with her father
- A mother who tells her 3-year-old daughter that she is a nasty child and that no one loves her
- A father who hits his 11-year-old son with a cane when he misbehaves
- A 13-year-old girl who can't remember the last time that her mother cuddled or kissed her

There is no right or wrong answer in Activity 15.10. All situations are different. How you feel about these examples will probably depend upon your own culture, values and beliefs. This is something that we need to respect and take into account for all the families in our care. However, it is important that you are able to recognise some of the clinical signs of abuse.

Activity 15.11

What factors would lead you to suspect that a child may have suffered the following types of abuse?

- Physical abuse
- Neglect
- Sexual abuse
- Emotional abuse

In your notes in Activity 15.11 you may have identified some of the following.

Physical abuse

- There may be physical markings on the child's body, such as bruising in unusual places, scratches, bites or cigarette burns.
- The family may have delayed reporting the incident and seeking medical attention.
- There may be a discrepancy between the child's physical signs and the history of the incident. For example, an 18-month-old child with scalds to both feet, which the parent(s) say was caused by the child stepping into a hot bath.
- A knowledge of child development may identify that a child could not possibly have sustained the injury in the manner described. For example, a 6-week-old baby may have bruises on the back which the parents say is the result of the baby rolling off the sofa. Babies of this age are unable to turn themselves!

- The child or sibling(s) may have a history of previous injuries that have not been fully explained. The family may also exhibit abnormal attitudes and behaviour – they may be over-protective of the child or, conversely, they may display little interest.

Neglect

- The child is likely to appear unhappy and may be withdrawn or aggressive, with lingering health problems.
- He or she may have problems at school, such as truancy.
- The child may look unkempt, with signs of poor care, for example failure to thrive and severe nappy rash.

Sexual abuse

- The child may act out sexual activities in role play with a teddy or doll.
- There may be soreness, bleeding or itchiness around the child's genital area; there may be signs of ano-genital trauma.
- The child may display sexual knowledge beyond his or her years.
- The child may exhibit fear towards a particular individual.
- The child may have a low self-esteem.

Emotional abuse

- The child is likely to appear withdrawn and nervous.
- Personality changes may be evident and the child may have difficulty forming relationships.

From these points it will be clear that in some cases it may be difficult to identify child abuse. Perhaps one of the most important first steps in recognising ill-treatment is to listen carefully and *believe* what the child is saying. Initial belief is especially important so that later questioning does not silence the child. Coupled with this, observation and accurate reporting of the child's activities are fundamental. The child may exhibit thoughts and feelings through drawing, poetry or play. It cannot be emphasised enough that the whole family needs to be assessed. If you are concerned that a child may have suffered abuse, discuss your worries with a senior member of staff immediately. Your response could dictate the future care and management of the child.

Caring for the child who has been abused – your own feelings

The thought of a child suffering any form of abuse may arouse very uncomfortable feelings within you. Remember that you are no different from anyone else and that it is natural for your emotions to rise. However, it is essential that you recognise these feelings and do not try to stifle them. Your own clinical area may have regular meetings or self-help groups, often facilitated by a psychologist, at which you may have the opportunity to explore your feelings. Alternatively, it may be appropriate for you to talk to one or more of your clinical colleagues who have also been involved in the child's care. Just airing your thoughts and views can help tremendously. Although child abuse is a widespread and worrying problem, you may never encounter a child who has suffered ill-treatment. It is important to remember that by far the majority of children are loved, wanted and cared for by their families. If you do suspect child abuse do make sure that your concerns are passed on to other specialised personnel who will be able to fully investigate the situation.

Summary

We have considered some aspects of the care of children in hospital. It is of paramount importance that the child and family are regarded as one in planning and providing care. A hospital visit can be potentially very traumatic for a child. However, as carers it is our responsibility to ensure that, for the majority of families, their transition from home to hospital and back home again is as smooth, safe and uneventful as possible.

Remember: A hospital stay can be a happy, positive experience for child, family and carers.

References

1. Bowlby, J. (1951) *Maternal Care and Mental Health.* World Health Organization, Geneva.
2. Robertson, J. (1958) *Young Children in Hospital.* Tavistock Publications, London.
3. Bowlby, J. (1969) *Attachment and Loss: Volume 1 Attachment.* Hogarth Press, London.
4. Shannon, F.T., Ferguson, D.M. and Dimond, M.E. (1984) Early hospital admissions and subsequent behavioural problems in 6 year olds. *Archives of Disease in Childhood* **59**, 815–819.
5. Morrison, L. (1997) Stress and siblings. *Paediatric Nursing* **9** (4), 26–27.
6. Ministry of Health (1959) *The Welfare of Children in Hospital. Report of the Committee.* HMSO, London.
7. Burr, S. (1993) Adolescents and the ward environment. *Paediatric Nursing* **5** (1), 10–13.
8. White, D. and Woollett, A. (1992) *Families: A Context for Development.* Falmer Press, London.
9. Murdock, G.P. (1965) *Social Structure.* The Free Press USA, Pumell Distribution Centre, Bristol.
10. Bond, J. and Bond, S. (1986) *Sociology and Health Care.* Churchill Livingstone, Edinburgh.
11. Bruce, T. and Meggitt, C. (1999) *Child Care & Education.* Hodder and Stoughton, London.
12. Packman, J. and Hall, C. (1998) *From Care to Accommodation: Support, Protection and Control in Child Care Services.* The Stationery Office, London.

13. Aldgate, J. and Bradley, M. (1999) *Supporting Families through Short-Term Fostering*. The Stationery Office, London.
14. Brandon, M., Thoburn, J., Lewis, A. and Way, A. (1999) *Safeguarding Children With the Children Act 1989*. The Stationery Office, London.
15. Department of Health (2001) *The Children Act Now. Messages from Research*. The Stationery Office, London.
16. Department of Health (2002) *Personal Social Services Statistics. Table B14. Finished Consultant Episodes, All Specialities by Age Group and Sex, Year Ending 31 March*. The Stationery Office, London.
17. World Health Organization (1984) *Health Promotion. A Discussion Document on the Concept and Principles*. World Health Organization, Copenhagen.
18. Bunton, R. and Macdonald, G. (1992) *Health Promotion: Disciplines and Diversity*. Routledge, London.
19. National Voluntary Council for Children's Play (1992) *The Charter for Children's Play*. Children's Society, London.
20. Play in Hospital Liaison Committee (1990) *Quality Management for Children. Play in Hospital*. Play in Hospital Liaison Committee, London.
21. Child Accident Prevention Trust (2002) *Child Injury Facts and Figures – 1999*. Child Accident Prevention Trust, London.
22. Department of Health (1989) *An Introduction to the Children Act*. HMSO, London.
23. Department of Health, Home Office, and Department for Education and Employment (1999) *Working Together to Safeguard Children*. The Stationery Office, London.

Further reading

Alderson, P. and Montgomery, J. (1996) *Health Care Choices, Making Decisions with Children*. Institute for Public Policy Research, London.
Bee, H. (1992) *The Developing Child*. 6th edition. Harper Collins, New York.
Bruce, T. (1996) *Helping Young Children to Play*. Hodder and Stoughton, London.
Corby, B. (2000) *Child Abuse. Towards a Knowledge Base*. 2nd edition. Open University Press, Buckingham.
Department of Health (1991) *Welfare of Children and Young People in Hospital*. HMSO, London.
Dimond, B. (1996) *The Legal Aspects of Child Healthcare*. Mosby, London.
Hall, D. and Stacey, M. (eds) (1979) *Beyond Separation*. Routledge and Kegan Paul, London.
Hall, D. (1996) *Health For All Children*. 3rd edition. Oxford University Press, Oxford.
Hobbs, C.J. and Wynne, J. (1996) *Physical Signs of Child Abuse: A Colour Atlas*. Saunders, London.
Jessel, C. (1990) *Birth to Three: Parents' Guide to Child Development*. Bloomsbury Publishing, London.
Moyles, J. (Ed.) (1994) *The Excellence of Play*. Open University Press, Milton Keynes.
Perry, J. (1994) Communicating with toddlers in hospital. *Paediatric Nursing* **6** (5), 14–17.
Pfeil, M. (1993) Sleep disturbance at home and in hospital. *Paediatric Nursing* **5** (7), 14–16.
Schaffer, H.R. (1998) *Making Decisions About Children*, 2nd edition. Blackwell, Oxford.
Sheridan, M. (1997) *From Birth to Five Years*. Routledge, London.

Books and videos (to aid a child's preparation for hospitalisation and medical procedures)

Action for Sick Children (1999) *Herbie's Hospital Heroes.* Action for Sick Children, London.
Amos, J. (1998) *Separations. Hospital.* Cherry Tree Press, Bath.
Hart, L., Impey, M. and Satin Silver, J. (1998) *Ben and His Amazing Puffer.* National Asthma Campaign, London.
Kimpton, D. (1994) *The Hospital Highway Code.* Macmillan Children's Books, Basingstoke.
Smee, N. (1997) *Freddie Visits the Doctor.* Orchard Books, London.
Videos produced by Action for Sick Children, London:
   A visit to Children's Outpatients
   Jane's Operation
   Coping With Hospital

Chapter 16

Community care

Frank Garvey and Joan Harding*

Overview

This chapter provides an introduction to community care. It will help you to identify circumstances in which care is given outside institutions/hospitals and to make some comparisons between the two. The relationship between carers and clients is explored, following which there is a brief description of the organisation of community care and the care team. Finally, the chapter outlines standards of care within care delivery.

Key words: Individuals; home; rights; care; privacy; guests/visitors; property; support; care team; standards

The community

Your community is a social organisation, which provides the setting for dealing with most of the needs and problems of your daily life. It includes local authority services such as housing, education and social service departments that are managed locally through elected councillors and funded through your council taxes. It also includes traditional first-line health services – primary health care such as general practitioners (GPs), district and practice nurses, health visitors, midwives, dentists, pharmacists and optometrists, all funded from the central government Department of Health. On some occasions care cannot be provided through primary health care services. In these instances, referrals are made to specialist community or hospital trusts. This level of service provision is termed secondary health care.

Care in the community

Care in the community is usually taken to mean packages of support for individuals within their community setting. It can mean care that is provided for a person of any age, living within his or her own family unit and supported by a range of professionals within the primary care team. Assessment of the needs of

*Contributor to the original version of this chapter in the first edition.

carers is basically an extension of the assessment of the client's needs. Remember the well-being of the family is centrally important to the care of the client. The needs can be wide ranging: some purely practical, for example, supplying a hoist for moving and handling. Others can be more complex – focusing on the emotional and psychological effects of caring:

- The loss experienced in watching the physical and mental deterioration of a loved one
- Coming to terms with having a child with a learning disability
- Guilt and resentment arising from being in some way incapacitated or within tight financial constraints due to ill-health
- The lack of leisure time for carers
- Feelings of guilt

Support can be given to the main carers – often the client's immediate family, through respite care. Respite care can provide either periodic breaks – through the client moving into a professionally run home, or where carers come into the home – domiciliary carers, giving the care normally provided by the family.

Care in the community can also refer to the support of groups of people – such as those within residential homes for people with learning disabilities, older people, those with mental illnesses or for children. Local authorities, voluntary organisations or private individuals usually run these types of care services. Nursing homes provide for people who require longer-term care and whose health needs are too complex to cater for within their own homes.

Other health provision is found in the community: midwifery services providing pre-birth or antenatal care and home birth support, health visiting, community learning disability teams, psychiatric health teams and elderly care teams. The local authority departments – education, housing and social services – have a duty to work in partnership with the NHS and the local communities to tackle individual and community health issues. These agencies are required by the Human Rights Act 1998 to demonstrate equality and fairness, irrespective of a person's ability, religion, culture or ethnic background.[1]

Activity 16.1

A useful learning aid in looking at the needs of a person is to take the first letters (called an acronym) of the following headings (**SPICES**):

Social (relationships, support networks)
Physical (obvious signs of ill-health/mobility problems)
Intellectual (how much insight has the person)
Communication (how able is the person to engage in two-way communication)
Environmental (what hazards could there be)
Spending (what financial factors could be involved)

Using the above acronym, write down all the factors that you think important to consider in supporting an older person with a recurrent chest infection living alone in a flat during the winter months.

Differences between care at home and in the community

If you have ever been within a hospital either as a client or visitor you will have noticed the number of staff on the wards with the variety of uniforms and roles, the noise, the smells and the routines which continue day and night throughout the year. Hospitals are bureaucratic organisations staffed by people with a variety of different clinical and administrative roles. The aim is to provide individual care to large numbers of people in an efficient way. Hospitals have an array of equipment, caring aids and facilities to hand in a very technological environment.

Hospitals can appear as impersonal places, with the hustle and bustle of so many people going about their daily work. While effort is made to ensure that people's dignity is maintained, it can be hard to always achieve – one only has to think of the commode being used within a ward setting! When in unfamiliar surroundings, within a large institutional organisation it can be much more difficult to have your choices realised. For some people it can be very frightening to stand up for themselves and they can feel disempowered and overawed in what is after all, a very strange environment – full of strangers!

As a community carer, you will have the privilege of being a guest within an individual's home – whether that home is their house or their personal room. You will be entering into an unwritten agreement of trust. You may be going into areas within a person's home that are not normally open to visitors. One can understand how anxious clients must be, especially with new carers. Communication provides the links within the chain of a relationship. By using cues from an individual's immediate environment, such as photographs, medals, furniture, you can help stimulate conversation that will be individualised and meaningful and will form part of your developing caring relationship. Remember the client and family members are all partners in the caring process – as such you should be working to promote that teamwork.

Activity 16.2

There is an old saying 'Treat as you would like to be treated' that has much value in all caring situations. The next time that you are providing care to a person imagine you are the client. Upon reflection, would you provide care any differently?

Recipients of community care

People now live longer and enjoy better health as more illnesses are treated successfully than ever before. However, increased life expectancy brings about an increased chance of long-standing or chronic illnesses. For example, many older people suffer from dementia. They also have an increased likelihood of developing anxiety and depression. Can you suggest any reasons for this?

Nine out of ten NHS clients are seen in primary care and it remains the gateway to secondary care, for example through GPs referring people to their local hospitals for specialist consultations. While a small number of people with mental health problems require hospitalisation, most are cared for within their community. Some people are being rehabilitated – enabling them to regain, in part or full, their independence that may have been impaired by illness or injury. People who have acute or short-term health care needs can also receive care within their home – more usually on a short-term basis, where a full recovery is anticipated. Some women choose to have their babies at home with support from women-centred services provided either from their local GP practice or from their local maternity facility. People with learning disabilities – some of whom previously lived within large Victorian institutions or asylums (places of safety) – are now predominantly living independently or within small group homes run by private and voluntary organisations or the local authority.

With ever-increasing advances in medical skills and technology, there is an increasing trend for much shorter hospital stays. Many patients who, in the recent past, would have required a recovery or convalescent period in a hospital ward, are now admitted, operated upon and discharged home within the same day. Early discharge into the supporting network of 'hospital at home' or intermediate care has provided a release of hospital beds for those people in need of longer periods of hospitalisation.

This growing trend emphasises the need for careful discharge planning from hospital to ensure effective communication occurs to engage the correct services at the appropriate time. In considering the details of care given to clients in the community many of the principles and procedures discussed in the earlier chapters of this book will apply, adapted to suit the individual client and the particular home circumstances.

Activity 16.3

Ask somebody whom you know who is over 50 years old, to recall when they were children. See if they can remember how long people stayed in hospital for routine operations, such as appendectomy or tonsillectomy. How does this compare with current trends within treatment times?

Nature of community care

The Secretary of State for Health oversaw the development of the Health Act 1999[2]. This Act represents a modernisation programme within England, enabling health services and social services to work together in partnership and co-operation. There has been a recent shift of political and legislative power, with the formation of the Scottish Parliament (1998), the Welsh Assembly (1999) and the Northern Ireland Assembly. Although the structure of the health service differs within these areas, the underlying marriage of social and health care remains a central component within care delivery.

Health authorities are required to work with local authorities, the public, local private and voluntary health providers, GPs and health care trusts to produce a community Health Improvement Programme (HImP). The HImP document, copies of which would be held in the reference section of your local library, is a three-year local planning strategy for improving health and health care in people's local communities. It reflects the health needs of individuals within defined geographical areas.

Activity 16.4

Compare the differences in 'health' that might be found within an isolated rural community and a rich suburban town in south-east England.

April 1999 saw the introduction of primary care groups (PCGs) in England (Fig. 16.1). The PCG, as the name indicates, is the primary health care organisation that provides for a local community and generally invests in strategies to improve local primary care services as outlined in the HImP. The PCGs also have the responsibility for managing budgets provided by the health authority which are used to purchase specialist health care provision. Examples of this are when people require psychiatric services, maternity services, children and adolescent health services, health services for older people, for the terminally ill and specialist services for people with learning disabilities.

PCGs are made up of GPs, practice nurses, district nurses, health visitors and the support and administrative staff across geographical boundaries. The government intends for all PCGs to become primary care trusts (PCTs). These are free-standing organisations, having more power to not only buy in community services, but also to employ staff to provide them. Another new initiative is the NHS Direct – a nurse-led 24-hour telephone information and advice service. Also recently formed are walk-in centres, where people can get immediate treatment for minor health problems or injuries.

Activity 16.5

Find out the name of the PCG or PCT to which your GP belongs.

Standards of care

The Care Standards Act 2000 brings together the regulation of service standards and education and training within social and health care.[3] It applies to a range of services including residential care homes, nursing homes, children's homes, domiciliary care agencies, fostering agencies and voluntary health agencies including private hospitals and clinics.

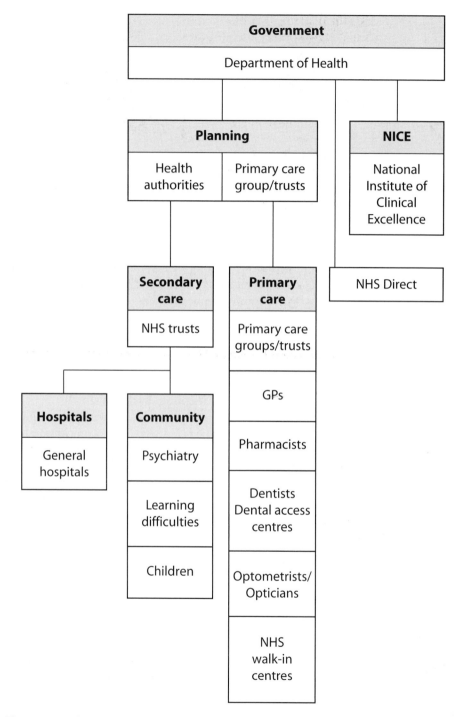

Fig. 16.1 NHS explained.

Since April 2002 care homes have had to comply with a range of new standards. The standards include sizes of rooms, completion of care plans, the support of individuals' rights, including level of personal choice, for example choosing what time meals are served. The Act also enforces that by 2005, a minimum of 50 per cent of 'care assistants' must be trained to NVQ Level 2. A new body – the National Care Standards Commission – will register and inspect care homes and the range of other services already mentioned to ensure that the new framework of standards is being met.

Within the PCG/Ts there is also a commitment to the improvement of care under what is termed 'clinical governance'. As well as measurement of performance against set standards, auditing, there is a need for NHS providers of health care to be able to demonstrate that care is based upon researched evidence that encourages best practice and professional development.

The National Institute for Clinical Excellence (NICE), an organisation directly accountable to the Department of Health, devises national standards for NHS care. These then form the framework upon which PCGs can deliver and monitor care. NICE also produce evidence-based programmes called National Service Frameworks (NSFs). These state exactly what people with certain health care problems can expect to receive from health care providers. NSFs have been developed for people with mental health problems, diabetes, care of older people and coronary heart disease and additional frameworks are being devised on an annual basis.

Summary

In this chapter we have looked at how individuals and groups of people within their community who require care are supported. In caring for another human being, the carer is required to look at the whole person in the context of their environment. It relies upon a partnership between health and social care with the client – delivering services that are based upon equality and fairness and are open to inspection. Care in the UK in the twenty-first century reflects the diversity of communities and their particular needs. Change appears to be the only constant – so fasten your belts!

References

1. Department of Health (1998) *Human Rights Act 1998*. HMSO, London.
2. Department of Health (1999) *Health Act 1999*. HMSO, London.
3. Department of Health (2000) *Care Standards Act 2000*. HMSO, London.

Further reading

Health Education Authority (1994) *Health and Lifestyles: Black and Minority Groups in England*. Action for Sick Children, London.

Royal College of Nursing (2004) *RCN Guidance on Professional Matters for Health Care Assistants and Nurse Cadets.* Royal College of Nursing, London.

Skidmore, D. (1997) *Community Care: Initial Training and Beyond*, 6th edition. Arnold, London.

Viner R. and Keane, M. (1998) *Caring for Children in the Health Services. Youth matters.* Action for Sick Children, London.

Useful websites

Department of Health Research and Development website: www.doh.gov.uk/research

NHS Confederation website: www.nhsconfed.net

Chapter 17

Caring for the terminally ill client and their family

*Angela Dustagheer and Elizabeth Atchison**

Death comes equally to us all, and makes us all equal when it comes
(John Donne LXXX Sermons, 1640)

Overview

In this chapter we will consider the care of the client who is dying and the care of the client's family and friends as they face their loss. We will also consider the needs of the carers, ourselves, for in learning about ourselves we will gain a clearer understanding of how to care for others. Different aspects of the support that might be given to clients and their families are illustrated in Table 17.1.

The term 'client' is used throughout this chapter in order to clarify the relationship between the 'cared for' and the 'carer'. The physical care of the dying client will not be covered in detail as this information can be accessed in other chapters of this book, e.g. hygiene, comfort, rest and other areas of care. We must always remember that the client facing death may need maximum amounts of care.

Key words: Culture; loss; grief; grieving; bereavement; beliefs; spirituality; religion; dignity

Culture

Clients requiring our care within the hospital or community settings are like all members of our society, people. People with their individual and very personal cultural beliefs: beliefs about illness and its treatment, about pain and about the entire hospitalisation or care process. Some of the beliefs will appear different, even unusual to us, as no doubt some of our beliefs will seem likewise to the client. We need to be conscious that what the client believes is not as important

*Contributer to the original version of this chapter in the first edition

Table 17.1   Dimensions of support for clients and their families.

Physical support	Psychological support
Spiritual and religious support	Social support

as the fact that they do believe it. Our behaviour to the client must reflect our understanding of the client's needs in this context.

If we accept that the individual's attitude to and acceptance of illness varies depending upon culture then we can begin to understand client differences. Some individuals express their anxiety, their fears and their pain freely, other people are more reserved. We must be very careful not to make rapid judgements in interpreting different responses, which are culturally determined. As an example we can consider how misinterpretation can occur when pain and its treatment needs are being assessed. Those clients who express their pain robustly may be identified as having lower pain thresholds than those who are more stoic or reserved.

Pain is what the client feels, any differences are in the way the individual client expresses their pain. In interpreting client behaviour we are making a judgement and when doing so we must try to remember to judge in 'the client's shoes'. That is, we must not say, 'If it was me this behaviour would mean I am angry, or hurt etc.', but we must say, 'What is the message I should receive from you?' Ask the client or family for more information before making judgements. The role of the competent carer is to treat the client's experience of pain with compassion, however the pain is expressed.

Loss

The experience of losing something is one which is encountered often in our lives. Many writers have suggested that the experience of loss is important to our development and that in working through our own losses we may more easily develop empathy with others. Certainly if we are aware of our own strengths and weaknesses in experiences then we may be able to relate more effectively to our clients. Lascelles suggests that it is much more difficult to cope with another's loss if we are still tied up in our own[1].

We need to be very aware of our behaviour when caring for the dying client and their families. Showing our concern and care is appropriate and is often a real comfort providing that it does not reduce our skills as a carer. 'There is no harm in crying with a client but it is not right to lose control'[1].

Considering loss further and our feelings towards it can assist our skills in caring. Loss can be of an object, a relationship, a part of the body, an organ or a limb, or of a person. Clearly some of these losses will threaten the well-being of the individual more deeply than others.

All loss, however, will lead to individual responses as people react differently. The nature of the experience of the loss and the support which individuals receive during it will influence how people cope with future life situations.

Activity 17.1

Think about an object of value you have recently lost. Note down your feelings at the time and your subsequent actions.

You may have recorded some of the following:

- Feelings – sadness, anxiety, panic, disbelief, anger, fear, shock
- Actions – searching, asking for help, going over your last steps, telling others or your family

Discuss these reactions with a friend or fellow carer and consider:

- How you responded as individuals
- Any differences you discovered
- How this exercise may aid you in caring for clients

The loss of some objects will be more significant than others and will influence the intensity and pain in the feelings of the loss. The greater the loss, the longer it may take for the individual to recover. Objects may not necessarily be of great financial value to be important to the individual but many objects are symbols of early or close relationships and their loss impacts greatly upon the individual who cannot replace them.

Feelings of loss are a unique experience. No two people ever feel exactly the same, although there is some common ground. Many variables can make loss more difficult to cope with including:

- The people we are, our previous experience of loss, the way we coped and the support available play a part.
- The circumstances in which the loss occurs, and our ability to make sense of it.
- The time scale of the loss: if we have time to prepare for a change we can accommodate leaving the past behind. If, however, we are suddenly parted from well known objects or possessions or people we do not have opportunity to take leave. Whether objects are relatively new or long-standing will also change the significance of the loss.

How does this knowledge of loss help us care for clients?

Activity 17.2.

List some of the losses which a critically ill or dying client or their family may experience.

You may have listed some of the following:

- Client – dignity, health, mobility, independence, appetite, weight, speech, role, taste, hearing, bowel or bladder control, vision

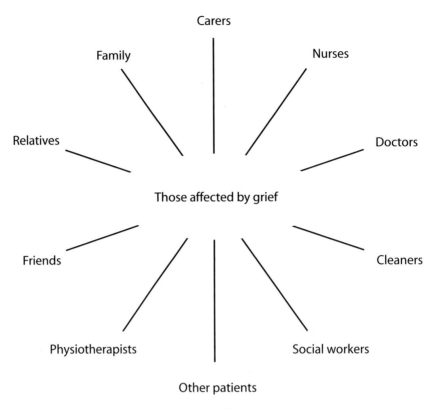

Carers

Family

Nurses

Relatives

Doctors

Those affected by grief

Friends

Cleaners

Physiotherapists

Social workers

Other patients

Fig. 17.1   Those who may be affected by grief following a death.

- Family – home, financial support, family member, soulmate, partner, lover, security, companionship, carer

Think of these losses when you next care for a critically ill client. Consider how you can adapt your care skills to respond to your client's needs and think how you can extend your care responses to your client's family and friends (Fig. 17.1).

The client's family and friends often play a very significant role during the client's illness. Communication with the family is very important. As carers we must be conscious how hostile the care environment can appear. It is often noisy and crowded and lacking in space and privacy. People need time to understand what is happening and to absorb the information being passed to them. If we can provide time and a quiet area for relatives so they can think, ask questions and absorb what is happening to them, this will help to ease their situation.

Bereavement

The death or imminent death of a loved person is the greatest loss an individual experiences. This loss is described as bereavement and the associated emotion as grieving or mourning. Many authors have described the emotions involved in grieving. Considering their views does not make the individual's situation less unique but can assist us to see common ground and so help us as carers to support clients. One such author is Elizabeth Kubler-Ross who said[2]:

> Those who have the strength and the love to sit with a dying client in the silence that goes beyond words will know that this moment is neither frightening nor painful, but a peaceful cessation of the functioning of the body.

In an effort to assist those caring for the dying person Kubler-Ross defined what she perceived as the stages people go through during or following the loss of a loved one. Other authorities refer to similar processes as 'defence mechanisms' or 'coping mechanisms'.

Kubler-Ross stages

There is no strict order and some stages run into each other or recur.

1. Denial: 'This cannot be happening to me.'
    Denial acts as a buffer, which gives time for the person to mobilise their defence mechanisms. It is very similar to a temporary state of shock. During this time the client or relative may talk of the future positively as if ignoring their prognosis. This is difficult for others to cope with.
    With time the individual will move to a state of partial acceptance.
2. Anger: 'Why me?'
    Often the anger gets displaced to family or friends or towards the hospital, the doctor or other carers. The individual's speech may become loud and their behaviour may appear aggressive. This is distressing for others if they do not understand what is happening.
3. Bargaining: In this stage the individual makes an attempt to postpone the inevitable. This often presents as a particular wish to do one last thing, to attend a wedding, to visit another country, play the piano once more. For some the bargaining is with God, 'If my child lives. . . .' or if I alter my lifestyle the overall outcome may change.
4. Depression: Now the individual feels numbness at the inevitability of the loss they are experiencing. It is unhelpful at this time to try to cheer up the person. The carer can assist best by allowing the client to lead the conversation and thus respond to their mood or just 'be there with them' in acknowledgement of their situation.

If the client can express sorrow in their own way then a degree of acceptance of their condition is easier.

Activity 17.3

Read the stages defined by Kubler-Ross[2]. Note the useful examples of how health carers can respond to clients in the different stages of grief, then discuss the issues raised with a friend or fellow carer.

Another authority who discusses the degree to which each person involved with a dying person will mourn or grieve is William Worden[3]. He wrote about the tasks those suffering loss might work through. Considering these tasks may help us as carers in the support we offer clients and families. The tasks of mourning are an attempt to move forward and to help both client and family to find life bearable again.

The tasks of mourning

To accept the reality of loss

In order to accept reality it is necessary to work through the issues of adjusting to the loss or impending loss (denial stage). This is a process which will take time. The client and the family may have many questions that need answers. The carer can help by listening and involving senior staff if there are questions they cannot answer. Family members may wish to re-visit the ward or care area following the client's death to check that their loved one is no longer there. This is a searching process.

To work through the pain or grief

Worden suggests that it is not possible to lose a loved one without feeling some emotional pain. This pain may be expressed as anger, depression, sadness, anxiety or fear. We cannot escape this pain; if ignored it will only emerge much later. The carer can help by being there for the individual and allowing them to express their feelings. If the individual becomes upset, it is the pain of loss which is distressing them not our presence. If the carer does not know what to say, be honest and express this – often just being there in thoughtful silence offers comfort.

To adjust to an environment in which the deceased is missing

This is a time of dealing with practical issues or of anticipating having to deal with practical issues, i.e. paying bills etc. Social or financial worries can cause great distress especially if those left have not been used to dealing with such matters. The carer can help by notifying senior staff who will contact other agents who may be able to help, e.g. social worker.

To find a safe place for the deceased in their emotions and move on with life

This state is achieved when the bereaved can cope with thoughts of the past and of the future. The loved one is not forgotten but life becomes bearable again. A time comes when memories can be received with a smile rather than tears. Perhaps at this point a new type of person emerges or a new stage in life commences.

Spiritual care

Our culture and experiences of life lead us to face death in different ways. Our aim as carers is to enable people who are dying and their families to feel that they are being cared for spiritually as well as physically. Often spirituality is linked with religious beliefs and followings but even those without religious beliefs tend to ask complex questions concerning their ultimate spirituality. Statistics quoted in the national press would indicate now that only a small number of people attend religious services in Britain and it is suggested that a larger number claim to believe in God and in some form of life after death. This is particularly so among older people. Conventional religions may not have a high rate of church attendance but many people have strong beliefs, which may manifest around the time of death.

Neuberger suggests that health carers will care better if they know something of the beliefs and traditions of clients and do not impose their beliefs upon them in the face of death[4]. This means familiarising oneself with some basic tenets of the beliefs of groups with which one comes in contact. In particular, an understanding of special needs concerned with the time of death will avoid the possibility of offending at such an emotional time. Often the only way to be sure not to offend is to ask.

Maintaining dignity

After a client dies it is the responsibility of the carer to maintain the dignity of that person, both for their sake and that of the family. The family may wish to be involved in the last care, often called last offices. Organisations have procedure manuals which document the conduct of these offices and carers should familiarise themselves with these practices.

Caring for the carer

This chapter has covered sensitive issues. This is perhaps the one area of care where one should think, 'How would I like it to be for my family?' to give a guide of how to behave. It may also remind us of feelings of our own losses.

We also face a grieving process and have an adaptation to make when a client for whom we have cared dies. We may have built a special relationship and may have learned a great deal from the way that person faced their death. In the situation where the primary carer is a family member, the sense of loss and sudden change can be devastating for them, especially where the 'routine' of care had produced a whole new life for those involved. Carers should be sensitive and supportive in the help they offer at this time. In may also be the time to call on one of the many organisations that help the bereaved, in the longer term, to understand and accept their loss.

Summary

We have briefly reviewed the areas of loss, grief and bereavement and identified some ways of dealing with these situations. We must remember that grief is a normal and necessary response to loss. The support of carers is vital for the client and their family. Carers are privileged to help clients and their families in a supportive way as they make the journey through loss.

References

1. Lascelles, R.V. (1991) *Coping With Loss*, 2nd edition. Pepar Publications, Birmingham.
2. Kubler-Ross, E. (1970) *On Death and Dying*. Tavistock Routledge, London.
3. Worden, W. (1991) *Grief Counselling and Grief Therapy: A Handbook for the Mental Health Practitioner*, 2nd edition. Tavistock, London.
4. Neuberger, J. (1999) *Dying Well: A Guide to Enabling a Good Death*. Hochland & Hochland.

Further reading

Akhtar, S. (2002) Nursing With Dignity: Part 8: Islam. *Nursing Times* **98** (16), 40–42.

Baxter, C. (2002) Nursing With Dignity: Part 5: Rastafarianism. *Nursing Times* **98** (13), 42.

Bowlby, J. (1980) *Loss*. Basic Books, New York.

Christmas, M. (2002) Nursing With Dignity: Part 3: Christianity I. *Nursing Times* **98** (11), 37–39.

Collins, A. (2002) Nursing With Dignity. Part 1: Judaism. *Nursing Times* **98** (9), 33–35.

Gill, B.K. (2002) Nursing With Dignity. Part 6: Sikhism. *Nursing Times* **98** (15), 38–40.

Khattab, H. (1993) *The Muslim Woman's Handbook*. Ta-Ha Publishers, London.

Lewis, C.S. (1961) *A Grief Observed*. Faber and Faber, London.

Neuberger, J. (1994) *Caring For Dying People of Different Faiths*. Mosby, London.

Northcott, N. (2002) Nursing With Dignity. Part 2: Buddhism. *Nursing Times* **98** (10), 36–38.

Papdopoulos, I. (2002) Nursing With Dignity. Part 4: Christianity II. *Nursing Times* **98** (12), 36–37.

Parkes, C.M. (1986) *Bereavement: Studies of Grief in Adult Life*, 2nd edition. Tavistock, London.

Saunders, C., Summers, D.H. and Teller, N. (1981) *Hospice: The Living Idea*. Edward Arnold, London.

Sheikh, A. and Gatrad, A.R. (2000) *Caring for Muslim Patients*. Radcliffe Medical Press, Oxford.

Useful addresses of care support agencies

Child Death Helpline

The Hospital for Sick Children
Great Ormond Street,
London, WC1N 3JH
and
The Alder Centre
Alder Hey Childrens' Hospital
Eaton Road, Liverpool L12 2AP

Cruse Bereavement Care

126 Sheen Road
Richmond, Surrey
TW9 1UR

PETAL (People Experiencing Trauma and Loss)

29 Clydesdale Street,
Hamilton, Scotland
ML3 0DD

Jewish Bereavement Counselling Service

PO Box 6748
London N3 3BX

Lesbian and Gay Bereavement Project

Healthy Gay Living Centre
40 Borough High Street,
London SE1 1XW

Winston's Wish

25 Clara Burgess Centre
Gloucester Royal Hospital
Great Western Road
Gloucester, GL1 3NN

Support for Carers

Princess Royal Trust for Carers
Campbell House,
215 West Campbell Street,
Glasgow, G2 4TT

Appendix
Cross-reference with NVQ/SVQ

Angela Dustagheer

This appendix cross-references the contents of the book with some of the units of competence as they appear in the National Occupational Standards for Care NVQ at Level 2. This book does not cover all of the available units for the award. It does contain some of the underpinning knowledge required for the four mandatory units (O1, CL1, CU1, Z1) as well as other units in Option Groups A and B. Each chapter is not a definitive work. Besides the reference list, further reading has been included at the end. It should be possible to locate the appropriate journals and books in any library within a university that has nursing courses, F.E. colleges that run health and social care courses and some public libraries.

NVQ Level 2 Units/Elements

Mandatory	Unit	Chapter
O1	**Foster people's equality, diversity and rights**	**1, 2, 3, 6, 10, 11, 14, 15, 17**
O1.1	Foster people's rights and responsibilities	
O1.2	Foster equality and diversity of people	
O1.3	Maintain the confidentiality of information	
CL1	**Promote effective communication and relationships**	**1, 4, 5, 17**
CL1.1	Develop relationships with people who value them as individuals	
CL1.2	Establish and maintain effective communication with people	
CU1	**Promote, monitor and maintain health, safety and security in the workplace**	**5, 9, 15**

Mandatory	Unit	Chapter
CU1.1	Monitor and maintain the safety and security of the work environment	
CU1.2	Promote standards of health and safety in working practice	
CU1.3	Minimise the risks arising from health emergencies	
Z1	**Contribute to the protection of individuals from abuse**	**1, 2, 5, 15**
Z1.1	Contribute to minimising the level of abuse in care environments	
Z1.2	Minimise the effects of abusive behaviour	
Z1.3	Contribute to monitoring individuals who are at risk from abuse	
Option Group A		
CL2	**Promote communication with individuals where there are communication differences**	**4, 5**
CL2.1	Determine the nature and scope of communication differences	
CL2.2	Contribute to effective communication where there are communication differences	
CU5	**Receive, transmit, store and retrieve information**	**1, 6**
CU5.1	Receive and transmit information	
CU5.2	Store and retrieve records	
Z6	**Enable clients to maintain and improve their mobility through exercise and the use of mobility appliances**	**7, 8**
Z6.1	Enable clients to exercise	
Z6.2	Assist clients to use mobility appliances	
Z7	**Contribute to the movement and handling of individuals to maximise their physical comfort**	**7, 8**
Z7.1	Prepare individuals and environments for moving and handling	

Option Group A		
Z7.2	Assist individuals to move from one position to another	
Z7.3	Assist individuals to prevent and minimise the adverse effects of pressure	
Z9	**Enable clients to maintain their personal hygiene and appearance**	**1, 2, 11, 13**
Z9.1	Enable clients to maintain their personal cleanliness	
Z9.2	Support clients in personal grooming and dressing	
Z11	**Enable clients to access and use toilet facilities**	**1, 2, 10**
Z11.1	Enable clients to access toilet facilities	
Z11.2	Assist clients to use toilet facilities	
Z11.3	Collect and dispose of clients' body waste	
Z19	**Enable clients to achieve physical comfort**	**1, 13**
Z19.1	Assist in minimising clients' pain and discomfort	
Z19.2	Assist in providing conditions to meet clients' need for rest	
NC12	**Enable clients to eat and drink**	**12**
NC12.1	Help clients to get ready for eating and drinking	
NC12.2	Help clients to consume food and drink	
Option Group B		
NC13	**Prepare food and drink for clients**	**1, 2, 12**
NC13.1	Enable clients to choose food and drink	
NC13.2	Prepare and serve food and drink to clients	
W6	**Reinforce professional advice through supporting and encouraging the mother in active parenting in the first 10 days of babies' lives**	**1, 2, 14**

Option Group B		
W6.1	Assist mothers to care for babies' safety, protection and security	
W6.2	Assist mothers in caring for babies' hygiene and well-being	
W6.3	Support mothers in feeding babies	
Z15	**Contribute to the care of a deceased person**	**1, 2, 13, 17**
Z15.1	Assist in the preparation of a deceased person prior to removal from the care environment	
Z15.2	Assist in the transfer of a deceased person to an agreed location	
Z16	**Care for a baby during the first 10 days of life when the mother is unable to do son**	**1, 2, 14**
Z16.1	Care for the baby's hygiene and well-being during the first 10 days of life	
Z16.2	Feed and interact with a baby	
Z8	**Support individuals when they are distressed**	**1, 2, 4, 17**
Z8.1	Contribute to the prevention of individuals' distress	
Z8.2	Support individuals in times of distress	

Index